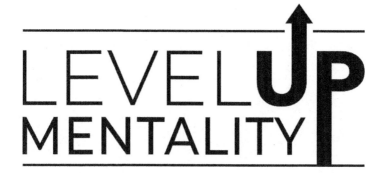

LEVEL UP MENTALITY

A Guide to Re-engineer
Your Mindset for Confidence

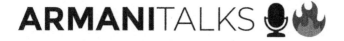

Table of Contents

The Author's Preface

The level up mentality is a lifestyle that can turn a rock bottom moment into chapter 1 of the greatest story ever. During our lifetimes, we are rarely taught the art of mastering the mind & mentality frameworks to follow. I want to change that & create a new reality.

For the past 5 years, I have worked as an engineer. And during my tenure as an engineer, I have been able to create, fix & enhance systems. It has been a wonderful journey to witness how engineering requires a breadth of creativity mixed with logic.

But as time went on, my focus went from working on physical products to researching the mind. When you look closer, the mind is not something that just exists, it is something that can be re-engineered. I thought the concept was ridiculous at first, but there was only one way to figure out. *Through experimentation.*

I decided to go on a journey to make sense of my past experiences & create a new reality. With engineering principles to stress test my concepts, practical systems analysis tactics & process design frameworks, I studied the mind.

Never had an engineer taken his talents to re-engineer the mindset. Was this a fool's wish or crazy enough to work?

Throughout the journey, I looked into limiting beliefs, subconscious reprogramming, how to build confidence and much more. I began to apply my concepts onto my own life.

After a few years had passed, my reality started to become very different. I went from a victim, to a victor. Went from unconfident to confident. Went from being shy to speaking in front of audiences of 500 people. What was happening? I know what it was. The mind was being re-engineered towards growth mode.

My theory about the mind being capable of being re-engineered was true in terms of my own life. Now the question was, how applicable were my frameworks to the world?

Since then, I have been sharing my mindset principles through my ArmaniTalks Twitter page, email list & website. On a weekly basis, I receive feedback as to how the practical concepts, mind hacks & level up frameworks have positively impacted many people from all parts of the globe. That went onto show that even if humans are all walking a different path in life, our minds have similar core concepts.

The mind is not a stagnant entity, it is a dynamic one. It is not fixed, it is capable of being rewired. Confidence is not something that we are born with, it is something that is exercised onto our existence.

My mindset framework to help you unlock growth mode & become your most confident self is known as **'Level Up Mentality.'**

The level up mentality deals with competing with your prior day self, building a north star for your life, designing an alter ego, skill building, leveraging emotional intelligence, optimizing social dynamics, chasing a legacy & much more.

This book is compiled of my top mindset principles, insights & practical tips. The best way to consume this book is to first read it from front to back to digest the concepts. Once completed, use it as a guide and come back to the sections which are most applicable to your life.

The level up journey will alter your mindset in many ways & will help you challenge prior limiting beliefs. But more importantly, it will add structure to a lost life & will push you to become your best self. If you are ready to delve into this journey, then let us begin.

- ARMANITALKS 🎙️🔥

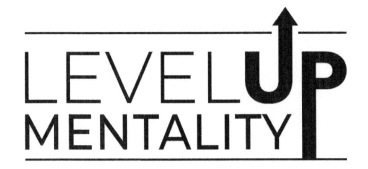

PART 1:
Darkness

The Story of Billy

A few years ago, there was a kid named Billy. Billy was in his mid-20s, had just graduated from college & was now working a job that he had no passion for. Billy was just showing up to life & hoping that things would eventually pan out. But unfortunately, it wasn't.

During his time feeling lost, he ended up going down a very dark path. This path consisted of him hanging out with a lot of losers, partying nonstop & learning the art of finger pointing.

You see, Billy did not understand why his life was the way it was. Why was it that he saw other people being happy with their lives while he felt so miserable? His resentment towards his peers grew & he wanted answers more than ever.

Was it the school systems fault?

No, it couldn't be that.

Was it his parents' fault?

No, not that either.

Was it the governments fault?

Hm, not quite sure.

Billy spent days & days looking to find the reason for his problems. Soon, those days turned into weeks & those weeks turned into months. Billy still hated his job, felt aimless & had nothing going on for him. He ended up going further down this black hole, until those months soon became YEARS.

Billy was trading in his golden era in exchange for being outraged. But what frustrated him the most was that he had no clue why he was so angry.

As years had gone by, Billy was slowly beginning to figure out what was going on. It wasn't until one of his later birthdays where he looked into the mirror, shocked at what he saw. At that moment, he had finally been given the answer that he had spent years searching for.

Billy came to realize that the only person who was responsible for his pathetic life was the person looking at him across the mirror.

The reason he had always felt empty was because he was looking for that next person to blame, rather than doing something about his situation. At this point, many of his friends had moved on up, had gotten amazing jobs that they loved, had a great family & felt happy with life.

Billy could not believe what he had done! How could he have been so stupid to trade in so many years with nothing to show for it? He had spent so many years going down this black hole that he would now have to spend the next few years digging himself out. A life of playing catch up. Sad...

Want to know a scary truth?

Level Up Mentality

Billy's story is far too common. Billy is your ideal victim. Someone who believes that their negative present-day circumstances have sealed a negative future. But why are there so many Billy's running around in today's world? I think I have a clue...

The Outrage Culture

Humans were born to solve problems, not get outraged by bullshit. But here's what happened:

*We live in the era of comfort; most humans don't have any **real** problems to solve.*

So what happens? Their brains create an ILLUSION of a problem to throw a hissy fit about. Sad way to live.

'Do these people know that they are seeing an illusion, not a real problem?'

Not at all.

'Why are they unaware?'

Because they are **brainwashed**.

Humans become brainwashed thru emotions. Once they control your heart, they control your brain. And this is a real threat to people without any real challenges.

'Any examples?'

Yes.

Level Up Mentality

-Look at the people on social media that hate on celebrities all day.

-Look at the people in the real-world whining about political scandals all day.

-Look at the people worrying about the opinions of strangers all day.

They don't have any real problems. They wouldn't know what a legitimate conflict was even if it walked up to them butt naked & smacked them in the face. So what do their brains do?

Their brains turn these scenarios which can easily be ignored, into HUGE threats. These people genuinely think they are in danger & there is no resolution.

Our ancestors would laugh at how soft the human population has gotten. They had to worry about getting eaten by a sabretooth tiger. And the clowns of our generation worry about the opinions & tweets of strangers they never met.

And the herd echo their sentiments to the world. They repeat & repeat their problems until other humans without any real problems pick up the same mindset as well. BRAINWASHING 101.

Thru this brainwashing, our culture has a herd of zombies running around looking for the next person to blame for their problems. This sort of thinking pattern has given birth to the modern-day victim.

Is Victimhood on the Rise?

For far too long, have you just been existing? Showing up to life & not sure what you are exactly doing? If this sounds strangely like you, then you need to be very alert.

'Why?'

Because if you don't create your identity, then it will be created for you. Society doesn't want self-sufficient winners. They want over consumers, victims & out of shape losers.

'Why?'

Because they are easier to control & profit from.

'Huh?? You sound like some sort of conspiracy theorist.'

No, this is all truth. It's time that you wake up.

'So you're saying society isn't actively pushing for me to become my best self?'

Correct. They want you to be subpar at best. Which is why they do a few things:

1.   They create a problem & sell you a solution.

2. They manufacture a problem to stir outrage & boost their ratings.
3. They shield you from the truth because most will be disturbed by what they see.

Don't you find it a little spooky that this is the GREATEST time in human civilization, yet the masses act like the world is about to end? It's because people don't know how to question the truth. They just blindly accept what they are told.

I'm here to tell you that you are being played. Society is actively trying to create your identity for you.

They want you to see race, not individuals. Which is why identity politics is glorified.

They want you to believe the rich is hoarding all the money, which is why you're broke. Vilifying success 101.

They want you to believe people who preach accountability, lack empathy.

This form of mental conditioning has led to an abundance of victims. People are being led to believe that they are a victim of their circumstances rather than a byproduct of their habits. With the rise of technology, it is easier than ever to spread negativity at scale.

Not sure if you know this, but the subconscious mind cannot distinguish between real & fake. This mind dictates 95% of your reality & views life thru images & emotions.

With the rise in technology, negative news, opinions & statistics are being spread at scale. This results in people feeling a lack of empowerment for their lives.

But let's be real, most victims have no clue that they are victims. You may continue reading this post and realize you were a victim all along. But where does this disease stem from? A few things, I'll just name a few:

1. **Coddling** - Kids who were coddled their entire life are the biggest victims. They think life is just supposed to be handed to them. But once they get out into the real world, they find out that's not how it works. Mom & dad aren't with you. But their soft mentality still stays the same.

2. **Mainstream Media** - Mainstream media has created a generation of weak, victim mentality clowns. These people genuinely think the world will end any second. Too brainwashed to understand they are being fed nonstop negativity for ratings.

3. **Repeat failures** - When someone fails the same way multiple times, it can do some damage. Many brush themselves off, analyze their mistakes, get 3rd party criticism and find a way to rise. But a victim? Exact opposite. They throw in the towel and decide that the system is rigged.

Signs of Victim Mentality:

Thinks life is happening to them

Uses past failures to justify avoiding future endeavors

Finger points

Level Up Mentality

Always blames a system

Lazy

Thinks all successful people are lucky

Has 0 vision

Amplifies the negatives and ignores the positives

Do You Resent Success?

At the core state, a human is a very emotional creature. A part of being an emotional creature is doing, feeling or thinking things that you often cannot explain.

Ask yourself this question, do you resent success? Many victims resent success, but never question WHY they resent success in the first place. They just feel the emotion of jealousy & then proceed to justify that emotion with misguided logic.

In the victim's mind, success is something that should be resented. When they see a successful person, a part of them automatically thinks 'privilege.' Were some privileged from birth? Sure.

But were all privileged? Absolutely not. That is simply a misconception due to a lack of perspective. Let me explain what many people who are privileged had to go thru:

Those 'privileged' successful people:

- worked a 40 hour a week job to come home and work some more on their dreams.

- weekends meant days to get more work done.

- they turned down numerous social events just for the sake of productivity.

- they chose books over TV.

- they chose themselves over their friends.

- they dealt with rejection repeatedly.

- they wondered if their vision was even worth chasing.

- they always came out of every conflict with poise.

- blood, sweat & tears to make their vision a reality.

While the victim was:

- pounding away alcohol in a pregame.

- pounding away more alcohol in clubs.

- displaying their drunk antics with pride on Snapchat.

- wasting their Saturday night doing the same thing that they did on Friday night.

- they do not remember any of the so-called memories they are creating.

- their Y.O.L.O mentality has morphed them from a free bird to a drunk sack of shit.

- then on Sunday, they reward themselves by watching Netflix and stuffing their body with garbage.

And instead of thinking 'hm may be my weekend warrior ways are setting my life back,' they do the **exact** opposite.

They make up this scenario in their head that the system is rigged against them. That they are not given opportunities in life. Then they assign a successful person the brunt of their blame. 'Look at this guy being successful. Wish I had his privileged life.'

But look closer! The victim wastes 3 out of the 7 days of the week. The successful person maximizes all 7 days to perfection. But that doesn't make a difference, right? The system is out to get them. Their boss and mom may to blame too, right? What a joke.

Resentment towards success will only ensure 1 thing: that you never achieve success.

Level Up Mentality

Now that you understand what victimhood is & why it exists, lets delve a little bit deeper.

What is the Comfort Zone?

The 2 Life Paths:

Path 1: short term pleasure for long term pain.

Path 2: short term pain for long term pleasure.

-Path 1 = Comfort Zone

-Path 2 = Growth Mode

The comfort zone is the byproduct of living a very easy life. You would imagine this to be a good thing. Comfort, what could be so bad about that? But the comfort zone is a very dangerous place to be stuck in.

You tend to get stuck into the comfort zone due to your subconscious mind. The subconscious mind is wired to seek comfort. Our primal ancestors were going out of their way to find food, shelter & safety in a very chaotic world.

But in today's generation, most humans do not really have to worry about that. We have food in our fridge, shelter over our heads & have safety on lock down. So, what next?

Level Up Mentality

Many decide all is good & decide to settle into the comfort zone. But here's the problem with settling. Our brains are naturally wired to tackle challenges. When it has no challenges presented, it will create its own.

When there is an abundance of comfort, our brains begin to blow small things out of proportion to turn it into a 'threat.' This leads to caring a lot about other people's opinions, getting offended quicker & skyrocketing anxiety.

Therefore anxiety is on the rise, even though we live in the most comfortable era in human history. With anxiety on rise, your life begins to feel a lot more clogged.

You begin to overthink, feel destructive emotions & think all hope is lost. This leads to a very negative viewpoint of life.

And understand this little psychological principle: *You project your internal world onto the external world.*

Picture yourself as a magnet. The energy that you are putting out there is the same energy that will be magnetized back to you. This concept is important to understand because it gives you a deeper understanding of victimhood.

A negative internal world gives birth to a negative external world. Then the negative external world causes a deeper resentment in the internal world.

That is how the comfort zone sparks a circle of toxicity.

Is Finger Pointing Becoming a Habit?

Finger pointing is the art of blaming your problems on another human. Finger pointing brings short term satisfaction in exchange for long-term powerlessness.

Every time, you finger point and blame your problems on another party, you will temporarily feel good because you have taken a load off burden off your plate. But the question is, who will solve the problem? The person you are blaming has their own problems to deal with, so they won't care if you are blaming them or not.

What you have now done is signal to your subconscious mind that you are not in control of your own life. That the problems you face is not due to your habits or actions but caused by a 3rd party. When you signal this command to your subconscious mind, you take away a great deal of your power and hand it over to someone else.

That is how the mindset of a victim works. They finger point on autopilot but lack the awareness to understand their behavior.

The opposite of finger pointing is **accountability**. Accountability is taking responsibility for the good AND the bad. Even if the bad was not your fault, you still take responsibility for it because it is your life & you are going to be the only one who deals with the negative emotions associated with the problem.

Accountability is when you bring on short term pain in exchange for longer term powerfulness. This is a lifechanging concept that will end victim mentality for good. But guess what?

A victim has their neural pathways too engrained to even give accountability a chance.

Why Group Thinking Is Dangerous

If you want to know the core difference between a victim & a victor, well, here it is:

The victor knows how to think for themselves & the victim opts to group think.

What is group thinking? Group thinking is letting the thought patterns of others dictate your thought patterns as well.

Now there is a time and place to be open minded & allow the perspectives of others to further enhance your mindset, sure. But group thinkers take it a level further. They literally rely on the group to think FOR them. That's when things begin to get dangerous.

This sort of herd thinking is dangerous because it makes a human dependent & an easy target for brainwashing. When you don't know how to operate one of the most powerful engines at your disposal, your brain, you tend to just wait for the group to reach a consensus so you can adopt that belief as well.

This level of dependency will have you overlooking opportunities & killing your confidence along the way.

Level Up Mentality

Everyone has had different experiences to get to where they are today. Using the experiences of someone else as the reference point for your own life will lead you to a lot of poor decisions & dangerous habits. Group thinking is a low social valued act that will have you acting like some extra in your life, not the main character.

How to Fix a Victim Mind

It's hard to fix a victim mind, not going to lie. You are basically rewiring years of structured neural pathways, limited beliefs & habits. But it's even harder because not only do you have to fix yourself internally, but you also must fix yourself externally. That's where things get difficult.

You typically won't see a victim surrounded by a bunch of victors. Victors are the types of people who take full responsibility for their lives. You will often see victims rolling with other victims.

Which is why negative thought patterns become reinforced, further sealing a reality.

Now even though victimhood is difficult to break out of, *it is possible*. And it traditionally happens thru 2 ways:

1. **Overtime**

2. **Rock-bottom**

The overtime strategy is when you are getting older, you are accumulating more experiences. And as you accumulate more experiences, you unlock new perspectives. The new level of perspectives brings in awareness to your life. Awareness is key if you want to disrupt limiting beliefs & negative habits. As you mature, your awareness helps you understand that you were the only one responsible for your life all along. It wasn't another person's job to get you what you wanted from your world, it was only yours.

The second option is the rock bottom moment. This is a moment that can happen suddenly and shatter a great deal of your world. Although this moment is much more painful than the prior process, it is faster. The rock bottom moment is an eye-opening time for many of us. If you have gone thru it in the past, then you know what I'm talking about. If you are going thru it right now, then read on.

The Rock Bottom Moment

Life has a funny way of humbling you. One thing that you will notice is that everything comes in peaks & valleys. You may currently be going thru a peak. You are in a committed relationship, have a dream job, drive a dope new car etc.

Life is going well & you seem to be on top of the world! You wonder how certain people out there don't have their shit together. What's so hard about managing your life? You just show up, put in the work & everything will be fine and dandy.

As you are living this dream life, out of the blue moon, something changes. Everything that you worked so hard for, comes crashing down before your eyes. Your relationship ends, you end up getting fired, and you crash your car.

A part of you feels like this is a nightmare that you will wake up from any second, that there is no way that your situation has gotten this bad overnight. Until you pinch yourself, feel pain, and realize that you are not asleep, you are awake.

Welcome to rock bottom.

The sudden or gradual downfall of your reality will be one of the most significant moments in your life.

After the event/s have transpired, you will feel broken within. Not only will you be out of it mentally, but physically as well. You are going to feel **extra** lazy. Your whole body is going to feel heavy & very warm. This may lead to excessive sleeping.

Other than feeling tired, you may lose your appetite as well. When I hit my rock bottom moment, I'd be lucky to even eat one meal day. Your lack of appetite will have you feeling even more lethargic. The lack of energy is going to make you spend more time in your head.

In order to escape your mind replaying whichever moment led to your rock bottom moment, you may turn to the bottle or the bong. You may believe that alcohol & weed will allow you to escape this nightmare. Will it? Sure. But only temporarily. However, once you are sober, same thoughts.

'Oh no! How long is this going to go on for?'

Depends.

'On?'

On you. Only you will be able to decide how long this spiral goes on for.

'So what do I do?'

You discover & rebuild yourself.

Here is the beauty about the rock bottom moment. You'll be the only person who pulls yourself out of it. Friends & family will help, sure. But ultimately, it will be your responsibility. You will be given 2 choices:

1. Stay in hell.

2. Engineer one of the greatest comeback stories ever.

Option 1 is the easy thing to do, because you just continue doing what you have been doing. And to be honest, most people choose to be a victim of their circumstances & stay in rock bottom. But this is a sad way to live because it impacts your present-day reality AND your future.

People who choose option 1 go on a downward spiral for weeks, months, or even years. One day, they see the people around them moving up in the world, accumulating value & building status. And when they look in the mirror, they see the same loser who has been moping around for ages. Once they make the realization that being a victim was never an optimal life choice, they are shattered.

They have wasted so much time that they will not get back. Now they have to play catch up on the game of life, desperately trying to clean up their past mistakes.

But that doesn't have to be you.

'How can I avoid this ill fate?'

By choosing option 2. By designing one of the greatest comeback stories ever. Ditch the life of the victim. Use your rock bottom moment to change your reality. Use this moment to make one of the best decisions of your life.

Level Up Mentality

If you are ready to become a victor, then you are ready to begin your level up journey.

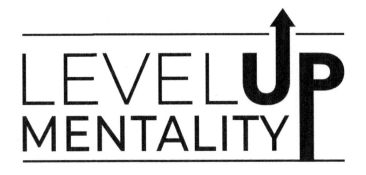

PART 2:

Level Up Journey

The Birth of a Winner

1. Spends years just existing.

2. Goes thru some traumatic event.

3. Struggles.

4. Breaks from within.

5. Introspects & rebuilds.

Time elapses...

6. The Phoenix rises from the Ashes.

The Winner is Born.

Amazing.

Writing Your Life Story

J.K. Rowling fought depression & was rejected by 12 publishers before her book series Harry Potter took off. Even if your life feels like a wreck right now, understand that it's never too late to change the narrative.

'But that's just J.K Rowling! How often do you see people switching up their life narratives?'

Too many times to count.

J.K Rowling is just one of many examples.

'Oh yea?'

Yea...

Jack Ma: Awful test taker, rejected from Harvard 10 times, turned down from multiple jobs. Heck! He was the only person from 24 people who got his KFC job application denied when the franchise was opening in his hometown. Yet, he still went onto discover the mega titan company, Alibaba.

Lebron James: His Miami Heat lost to the underdogs, Dallas Mavericks in the 2011 finals. The loss tarnished his reputation in the league & traumatized him. But he did not give up. He just worked harder & stayed true to his skill. Eventually, Lebron went on to win 3 NBA championships.

Walt Disney: He was fired because his boss told him that he lacked imagination. But he still stayed true to himself, kept his chin up & put in the work. Walt went onto win 59 academy awards & discover the legendary Disneyworld.

Colonel Sanders: We love KFC, but how many of us know its history? Mr. Sanders at age 62 was rejected by 1000+ people on his restaurant idea! But did he give up? No. He kept hustling until he was presented an offer. KFC is now a worldwide phenomenon.

'So I can improve even if I was a fuck up in the past?'

Sure. You are lowkey in an advantage.

'Wait, really?'

Yea.

-Bad experiences + Introspection = Wisdom

-Wisdom + Present = Clarity for the future

Leverage your past to your favor, your story is just beginning.

'My story is just beginning?? You mean I have a second chance?'

We all have a second chance, it's called **tomorrow**.

The Life of a Phoenix?

The Phoenix is a bird from Greek mythology most well known for being born again. After dying from being burned alive, the Phoenix was able to rise from the ashes & begin its new life.

You want to know something? Humans are capable of the same rebirth as well. If you are someone that is going thru a rock bottom moment right now, understand that your story is not over, it is just beginning.

Even if you were a fuck up in the past, you can turn your entire narrative around today. Even if you were a victim in your past life, you can begin the journey to becoming a victor today.

In order to become the Phoenix, you need to recondition your mindset towards a dark past.

There are 2 ways to view your past:

-Roadblock

-Speedbump

Roadblock: Many people who hold onto the past fall into this mindset. They feel like their negative past has sealed their fate. Their mind has created an invisible roadblock that will not allow them to grow. They hold onto the guilt & shame day in & day out.

Speedbump: This group of people has their eyes FORWARD. They focus on the entire picture of life, not just the pixels. Therefore, they realize their past mistakes were just speedbumps in their journey, not a life sentence.

In order to properly leverage your past, you need to go from:

Roadblock mindset -> Speedbump mindset.

To make the transition, you must understand that every human has a story. Some worse than others, but the story is present, nevertheless. The only difference between the winners & losers? The narrative they CHOOSE to assign to their story.

The losers CHOOSE to wallow in regret of their negative past.

The winners CHOOSE to make sense of their negative past.

One group leaves with more regret.

One group leaves with wisdom.

Those that have faced darkness & hardships in their life will always be at an advantage over those who have had a sheltered life. That's because in order to pull yourself out of darkness, you must have fight in you. And the more fight you have, the stronger your mind becomes.

-The arrow is pulled back before it is propelled forward. The farther it is pulled back, the more it propels. Same with life. The more darkness you overcome, the more you grow.

That's how you turn a bad situation into a breathtaking one. It all begins with the mind & the narrative you CHOOSE for yourself. You can either be the victim of your past or the victor of your future. But you can't be both.

It is never too late to turn your life around. I used to get suspended, was an awful student, had no clue what I wanted to do for my future & much more. But I turned my story around when I begin learning from my failures. So can you.

Look around you...

You think the people that are driven to succeed were always like that? Nah. Ask them. Pretty sure they had a period in their life where they were lazy & aimless. Then, after a long time of feeling lost, they decided to do something about it.

'So I am not broken? There is still hope for me?'

Yes, there is. Your drive is the most crucial component for your success. And in order to have drive, you need something.

'What?'

Fire.

'Okay! Let me buy a lighter from 7/11 then!'

No silly, I mean the fire from within.

'Huh?'

The fire within you is something that radiates in your heart. That energy allows you to achieve your wildest dreams.

'Which YouTube video can I watch to get that fire?'

None.

'Any resources?'

Yes, yourself.

Fire is often crafted from pain.

'I thought it was formed from wanting a better future?'

Sure, that will work for some. But for me and many others, we formed our fire thru pain. We felt hurt, shame, & disappointment first hand. We were lazy bums in our past life. So what did we do? We did something about it.

As our friends & families were making something of themselves, our jealousy grew. Instead of using our jealousy to hate, we used it as a compass. We found out exactly what made us jealous & decided to chase it.

Whatever pain it is, use it to your advantage.

Pain is simply energy that can serve as your battery for growth.

Level Up Mentality

Pain is your missing puzzle piece to greatness.

Pain is something that a book will never give you.

It is something life experience will deliver you.

Handle it like a warrior.

Once you have the fire, something beautiful will happen. You have unlocked a new level. Your whole life, you only thought with your brain, but you didn't know how to feel. You didn't know diddly squat about your gut, instinct & intuition. But the fire connects you to all of that.

2 things that you need to succeed: **Brain & Heart.**

Picture yourself driving.

Brain is the steering wheel.

Heart is the gasoline.

One cannot work without the other. Well, it can... but you will be mediocre. We are going for legend or bust, so you NEED both.

If you are feeling lost, do not give up yet. You need to feel lost in order to find the right way. Believe it or not, being lost is part of the process in the journey towards greatness. You are simply in the beginning chapters of your story. You just need to keep on writing.

As you are writing, you will notice that each chapter is making more & more sense. Don't you see what is happening? You are in the process of writing the greatest story EVER. Every book needs a conflict, but every hero always finds a way to overcome. You are no different.

From here on out, your life is a story. View your past as Chapter 1. You are the author & protagonist. The narrative, settings & characters are within your control. Overcoming conflicts & challenges are what keeps your story entertaining.

Now you are ready to adopt Level Up Mentality.

What is Level Up Mentality?

Level up mentality = Competing with your prior day self for the rest of your life.

Although this may seem like a daunting mental shift to make, it will help you become your best self. Adopting this mentality is how you become the mythical Phoenix who is reborn.

Adopting level up mentality will allow you to engineer your future.

For most of your entire life, you have been taught to compete with others, resenting what they had & undervaluing what you had. But where did that get you? It may have helped you grow in certain facets of your life, sure. But incessant competition with others does not make you better, it ultimately leaves you feeling empty. Adopting the level up mindset hacks your brain into growth mode while unleashing your happiness in the process.

Traffic Jam vs. Clear Lane Mindset

Competing with everyone gives you a traffic jam mindset. Competing with your prior day self gives you a clear lane mindset.

Let me explain the differences between the 2 perspectives so it will make sense why you are adopting the level up mentality.

Competition with everyone: this is when you are creating endless competition. You are simply inviting traffic into your life.

'So ditch my competitive spirit?'

Hell no! You need that. But let's redirect the competitive spirit. I will come back to the redirecting concept shortly.

Competing with others has your ego being pulled in too many directions. Very poor strategy for long term growth. Want to know something? When you compete with others, you don't get better, you get bitter.

'Why more bitter?'

You become more bitter because you never celebrate shit. Say you got 1000 YouTube subscribers on your first month. Impressive feat, right?

'Yes.'

Well, your mind will immediately hop off that accomplishment to find someone who got 2000 subscribers in a month. Instead of being happy, you find a way to poke holes in your accomplishment.

Realize that everyone is on their own path. Comparing your 3-month self to someone else's 3-year self is misguided & foolish. Your stacking up accomplishments with the sole goal of beating other people. What kind of journey is that? You invite unneeded traffic into your life.

But what about if we want to see a clear lane?

Competition with your prior day self: Now instead of trying to beat everyone, you are *inspired* by them. You immediately replace your bitter negative emotion with a positive empowering emotion. You have replaced a shitty battery with one full of life.

With the new battery, you are more energized than ever. Your mental clarity & emotional state is now working WITH you & not against you. It's time to leverage that inspiration to make significant life changes!

'Example please?'

Glad you asked.

Say you are trying to grow a Twitter following. See what other successful people on the platform consistently do, day in and day out. Then, simply incorporate some of their strategies as well. That is how you get inspired like a boss.

'What about my competitive spirit?'

Remember how I said we were going to redirect your competitive spirit?

'Yes.'

Well now you are competing with YOU. From here on out, you want to always outdo your prior day self. That is your **only** competition. Your prior day self is a bum & must be defeated at all costs.

Get it?

1. Grab strategies that inspire you to grow & use your own strategies.

2. Implement.

3. Make today better than yesterday & tomorrow better than today.

These 3 principles are the core fundamentals of the level up mentality. This is how you HACK your mind into growth mode.

And the most beautiful part? You are now running your own race, not someone else's.

This mentality shift will make you go from a bitter dud -> better stud. All the cars are gone now champ. No traffic at all. The highway of life is all yours. The world is yours. Just drive forward EVERY day. You can stop to fill up gas, but don't ever stop driving!!

The level up mentality shift will change your life for the best.

Using Forgiveness to Level Up

Forgiveness is a prerequisite to letting go. Letting go is a prerequisite to moving on. Moving on is a prerequisite to growth.

'Why does life feel so difficult?'

Because you're holding onto guilt & 'what if' scenarios. You need to forgive yourself.

1. Make amends with your past.

2. Have clarity for the present.

3. Manifest your dreams of the future.

Bingo.

Holding onto guilt will only result in more guilt. We often do this without even knowing that we are.

Picture this.

You are running a race.

53

But you are running it with an anchor tied to you.

Can you run the race at full speed?

No, you can't.

Same with life, picture this.

You are *trying* to level up.

But you are doing it with regret, guilt, doubt & what if scenarios.

Can you progress at full speed?

No, you can't.

You are quick to forgive others, but you are slow to forgive yourself. Why?

'Because I feel like I don't deserve forgiveness.'

But you do, we all do.

However, there is a catch.

'Which is?'

You need to LEARN from the mistakes first.

Because everyone deserves forgiveness, but only a few will *earn* it. Let me explain.

54

Humans are flawed creatures. We make mistakes & have lapses in judgment. But humans are adaptable creatures. We have the capability to evolve.

You evolve by using your past as data. No point in going thru an experience if you are never going to learn from it. Your past will give you wisdom that will last for another 10 lifetimes. You will one day see that regrets lead to growth. Regrets serve as your **compass** on where to introspect:

Regret + Introspection = Wisdom

And that is how you make amends with your past. You learn from what you did right & what you did wrong. By doing both in harmony, you will evolve.

Once you begin evolving, the anchor that you were running with becomes lighter & lighter so you can run faster & faster.

You now have clarity for the present-day. And the present-day clarity allows you to develop a laser-like focus for your future.

It all begins with learning from your past mistakes & forgiving yourself. Until you do that, your level up journey will feel like mission impossible.

But once you forgive yourself? Life will no longer feel difficult, it will feel fulfilling.

And that is how you leverage your past rather than letting it self-destruct you. That is how you turn the anchor into fuel. Once you have done that, you are ready to level up to unprecedented levels.

Leveling Up Requires Selfishness

The level up mentality requires a:

-selfish -> selfless transformation.

You need to be very selfish to fully love yourself, the good & the bad. Once you love yourself, you become confident. Next, be selfless & help others love themselves.

Where many people go wrong is that they flip this strategy. They are too selfless in the beginning stages.

'What's wrong with being selfless?'

It's a poor strategy when you have yet to discover your own value.

'Hmm...not sure I'm getting what you're saying.'

When you do not value yourself & simply try to make others feel valued, something dangerous happens.

'What?'

You approach life as a low social valued person. This will negatively affect your mannerisms.

'Affect it how exactly?'

You'll begin doing stuff like:

-Giggling a lot

-Agreeing non stop

-Displaying uncomfortable body language

-Speaking softly

-Avoiding eye contact etc.

Sound familiar?

'Yes, seems like you're describing a nice guy.'

I am.

Niceness happens when someone wants to make others feel valued without even valuing themselves. Results? The other person treats the nice person like a low social valued person. This is a very sad thing to witness, especially considering the nice person means no harm.

Which is why I recommend the selfish to selfless strategy. I always put myself unapologetically first. I'm always looking out for my best interests above everyone else's and I feel no shame for doing this because I do so with good intentions.

'How? Seems like you're being selfish.'

I am.

At the 'selfish' stage, you are aiming to become the best version of yourself. You ruthlessly chase whatever your life vision is & continue to cross off your goals. Each goal you cross off, the more your value rises. Let me solidify this concept with an analogy.

Which pilot do you want flying your plane?

A. The person who took a few flight classes before dropping out.

B. The person who completed flight classes & successfully flew a plane a bunch of times?

'B of course!'

Why?

'Because B has more experience & value.'

Exactly! The fact of the matter is that A and B both may have good intentions. But B can actually help people because they have put in work to be valued. And now you must do the same. No point in helping others if you are going to provide a subpar version of yourself.

Take the time to invest in your life & be selfish. Become the best version of yourself that you can be. Once you feel like you are gaining skills & starting to value yourself, THEN you can be selfless. And trust me, people will love you more for it!

Level Up Mentality

Once you begin helping people, you will be able to identify a lot of the problems they are facing. Why? Because you went through those same problems first hand in your selfish stage! Which is why you will be able to provide super precise tips & tactics to help them overcome their own shortcomings

The fact that you are helping people with their flaws makes them realize that they are not alone. In your selfless stage, you are guiding people to become their best self. Results? They soon begin to love themselves more. You will inadvertently be seen as a charismatic star.

That's how the game was meant to be played. Adopt the selfish to selfless lifestyle today. You will grow & help others grow in the process.

2 birds with 1 stone.

Leveling Up
REQUIRES Accountability

People who practice accountability are hard to control. They know how to think for themselves. Society doesn't want that because people who think for themselves are the first ones to break the norms that society has set for them.

How often do you see the mainstream encouraging people to be accountable for their own lives? Rarely, if ever.

What you see from the mainstream is limiting beliefs being pushed nonstop. They push tons of these narratives that say that your skin color, age, gender will prevent you from having the life that you want. Victimhood 101.

Pure bullshit. My family & I came from the villages of a 3rd world country, came to the US & dealt with our fair share of discrimination. But guess what? We still rose. How? Thru **accountability**.

We knew that bitching about our circumstances would get us nowhere. So, we worked on our English, found jobs, made connections etc. We overcame each obstacle that was thrown our way.

Level Up Mentality

And as we became more accountable for our lives, our ability to think for ourselves grew. We started to see thru the propaganda that society has been brainwashed by.

Your circumstances were never the problem, your weak mind was.

But society wants weak minds running around mainly because weak minds are easy to control. Accountability changes up the ENTIRE game. Accountability forces you to exercise your mindset by taking responsibility for your own damn life. That's how you discover your inner power.

It's been 20+ years since I moved to the US. Since then, I've run profitable ecommerce stores & marketing campaigns, worked on a patented device, am an engineer etc. While many others that came to the country around the same time are still blaming their skin color for their problems. Laughable.

Finger pointing & being a victim is nothing to be prideful of. It's something to be ashamed of.

Don't fall for the trap of getting brainwashed. You have *full* control over your life.

Which is why being accountable is a staple of the level up world. You need to take the blame for ALL of your problems and your brain WILL search for solutions, guaranteed.

When you take responsibility, it awakens the hidden beast within you. Your subconscious mind hates to be in danger, so it starts working in overdrive to get you to overcome the threats. That's the power of your mindset.

As you keep leveling up, accountability becomes your safe haven. You realize that the world is super volatile & unpredictable. But the only thing that you will always have control over, are your actions.

Control over your actions leads to control over your results.

Control over your results = Control over your narrative.

Control over your narrative = Empowered mindset.

Get it? You spark a chain effect of growth when you make it a priority to be accountable for the good AND the bad. Once you do, your mindset will begin to exponentially grow.

That's how you play chess while everyone else plays checkers.

Chasing a Legacy

You never know who you are secretly inspiring. Just put in work for your given field, stay humble, show results & you will have unknowingly formed a tribe.

Before you commit to the level up mindset, I want you to ask yourself, what is the end goal?

If it's just to improve to get yourself out of darkness & then go back to your old ways, then this may not be the right mindset for you.

Emotions are temporary. So if you are feeling out of it due to your rock bottom moment, then understand the feelings will one day go away. But when the feelings go away, what next?

Going back to your past self as a victim will not make this a valuable journey. All you are doing is leveling up to eventually level back down. Picture a person who goes on a journey to lose weight, hits their target goal, then gains all the weight back. Pointless if you ask me.

But if you are going to consistently push your ceiling even when the dark emotions go away, then level up mentality is for you.

The main purpose of level up mentality is not to make a couple of extra bucks, get in shape, or design a cool blog. The main purpose of level up mentality is to create a legacy. Your goal is to become a legend.

But isn't being a legend too difficult? Not quite.

A legend is seen as someone who has positively impacted the lives of a certain group of people. Note, I did not say the entire world, I said a certain group of people.

Your ultimate purpose of leveling up is to chase a **north star** which enhances you to grow at significant levels. As you grow, you will then be called to give back. You can give back to your parents, kids, or community. Whatever it is, you must give back.

You need to positively influence the lives of a few other people in this world before you take your last breath, otherwise, you did not properly do your job.

We are going for legend or bust when we adopt level up mentality. The losers will automatically admit to defeat & give up here.

But the winners? They are ready to proceed onto the next step, because they know that they have a primal desire to give back. It's time to turn your rock bottom moment around & level up for life.

Let us begin.

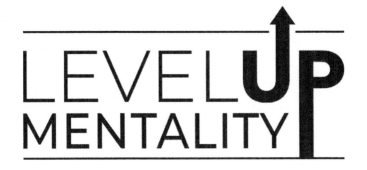

PART 3:

Creating Your North Star

The Importance of a Life Purpose

You are not born with a purpose, you cultivate it.

The level up journey requires a north star. Without it, you are just aimlessly walking around in circles. When you don't have a life purpose, you will often be wasting your time & not even know it!

It is very important to have a life purpose due to how the brain operates. The brain thrives off challenges, conflicts & most importantly, a **mission**. When you fail to assign your brain a mission, it will assign one for you.

This is risky because your brain may not always give you the best mission that suits your desires. When you fail to assign yourself a life purpose, your brain will begin to blow small things out of proportion. You will notice yourself:

-Caring about opinions a lot.

-Feeling excessive boredom.

-Feeling a high level of anxiety.

These are just a few side effects of not having a purpose. When you don't seek challenges, your brain seeks them out for you.

Which is why, instead of walking in circles all day, I want you to design 1 path with a north star at the end. The north star will be hazy at first, but it will clarify the more you walk forward on your path.

With the north star in your life, you are making an effort to take steps forward everyday which will tremendously simplify your life. When your life simplifies, you no longer give any energy to drama, haters, snakes, getting revenge and all that other noise.

You become much more selective with your attention & begin investing your energy into leveling up.

Now that you understand the importance of the path, let's help you design one.

Designing a North Star

People who actually care about what they're doing have a different glow to them. They have energy, drive & a positive spirit that will brighten up your day.

'I've noticed that glow too! Why is that?'

It's because they have reached internal harmony. When the harmony is there, magic happens.

In order to reach harmony, your brain AND heart need to align. When one is off, you will not feel right:

-When your brain is in it, but your heart is not:

This will feel like work. And when something feels like work, you tend to drag your feet. You may get the task done, sure. But with 0 enthusiasm.

-When your heart is in it, but your brain is not:

This will feel like confusion. You'll have a lot of fun, but something will feel off. You keep wondering how this act will help you move forward in life. You wonder if you're being childish.

If you are someone getting started on your journey, you may have no clue where to begin. I know I sure didn't.

'What did you end up doing?'

I went on a journey to discover my journey.

Finding a purpose & reaching harmony is **earned**. So, you will not reach it from the beginning. You will run into many activities that are not harmonious & begin to doubt yourself.

In order to find the right activity for your life, you will often take 2 different paths:

1. External - Someone from the outside world has identified what you should be in life. Many times, parents may fall into this category.

Example: a lot of people want their kids to be doctors. Results? Your purpose is identified for you.

2. Internal - This is the one I will expand on a little more on. At this point in your life, you feel lost because you may not have reflected enough or do not have enough experiences.

You got to this point in life by going thru your fair share of experiences. Question is, how often do you reflect upon it to extract the lessons? If you can't think of the last time you reflected, then you may have already experienced what your life purpose should be, but you haven't bought awareness to it. Reflect on your past experiences & make sure that you are not overlooking evident answers.

However, if you are someone who hasn't experimented much with life, then you need to experiment! How are you going to identify your target without any data?

'So what do I do?'

You ever had a gut instinct?

'Yes, of course.'

That is your body trying to tell you something.

'Okay.'

You ever had a curiosity?

'Yes, of course.'

That is your mind & soul trying to tell you something.

'Whoa!

Which is why I recommend you follow your gut & curiosity in the initial stages. When you have a scratch, you need to itch it. Finding your purpose will often require you to take some risks. A lot of times, your gut & curiosity will point you in a scary direction.

'Why is it scary?'

Because you are delving into the unknown, which is why you need to show courage. You'll never know if it was meant for you if you don't try it.

'What if I fail?'

If you fail, then you fail. But at least you got your lessons & data out of it. That's the most important part.

As you are approaching these activities, you need to keep 3 things in mind:

1. Patience

2. Creativity

3. Consistency

1. **Patience:** Every new activity is hard in the beginning. But you need to pass thru the hard stages to form an honest opinion. If you just quit because it's tough early on, you're potentially losing your life altering activity! PATIENCE.

2. **Creativity:** In order to be patient, you need to be creative. Find unique ways to make the hard stages fun.

3. **Consistency:** Keep being consistent & you'll pass thru the hard stages. The difficulty begins to melt away. When the difficulty melts, then you can form an honest opinion.

'Isn't that a lot of work?'

Level Up Mentality

Sure. But who said finding a life purpose was going to be easy? But I have good news for you.

1. Finding your life purpose = hard.

2. Going all in on your life purpose = easy.

So you're going thru the hard part now. But once you find out what works for you, everything becomes easier!

Reaching harmony makes you feel like you're never working a day in your life. You're just doing what you love. Your life becomes colorful & full of meaning.

Soon, you'll have energy, drive & a positive spirit that no one can ever take away. With that being said, find your harmony activity & don't stop till you do!

Create a Desire

-Burn back up plans

-Put images of your goal in your environment

-Speak your future into existence every morning & night

-Surround yourself with driven people

-Set deadlines

-Take action until your mind goes from thinking -> knowing

Questions to Discover your North Star

Ask yourself questions that you seek the answers to. You'll awaken the creative side of your brain. It will call on your neurons to find the answers. Then, you will get flashes of the answers when you least expect it. Aka: Epiphanies. Magic.

'What's up with the hocus pocus shit Armani?'

Far from it, my friend. Have you ever had that moment when you were trying to recall something, but you couldn't? You thought & thought, but nothing?

'Yes.'

So you gave up thinking and went back to your day.

But as time elapsed, out of nowhere, the answer popped into your head. You had your eureka moment!

Well, this same concept is applicable to other facets of your life. It just comes down to understanding your 2 minds.

The 2 minds:

-Conscious mind: your critical thinking mind. The tip of the iceberg.

-Subconscious mind: the database of your entire life. The iceberg.

Questions make your conscious & subconscious mind work together. When you ask a question with your conscious mind, your subconscious mind has the urge to answer it. And it will not stop working behind the scenes until it does.

1. Ask detailed questions that you seek the answers to. Be vivid & ask questions that make you feel. Think BIG.

2. The subconscious mind will awaken & get to work.

3. Await the answer.

The answer can come to you at any random time. Often, you'll be presented with the answer & just brush it off because it's not logical. But don't! The airplane, light bulb & phone were all seen as illogical, until it was not.

Humans have more power than we give ourselves credit for. We can turn the impossible to possible if we have the desire to do so. Don't sleep on your potential.

Ask yourself questions as you are going thru your experiences, and you'll notices flashes of answers coming to you. That's how you wake up your inner Houdini.

3rd Perspective Yourself

Tame your ego & think: 'Would I want to hang out with myself?' Be honest. If not, find out why. Once you have identified the reasons, fix those flaws & quirks. Simple. That is how you audit your personality.

'Why not view my flaws thru 1st perspective?'

Because you are leading with your ego. Leading with your ego may have you overlooking flaws that are holding you back. Therefore, you need the 3rd perspective strategy to momentarily kill your ego.

Go on, close your eyes & see yourself coming up to you.

Friendly face or angry face?

Good vibes or bad vibes?

Polished or sloppy?

Keep analyzing.

Doing this strategy will give you a lot of wake-up calls that will help you navigate towards a north star. The beauty about this strategy is that it brings awareness into your life. You will have no clue what to change or level up on if you have no clue what to change or level up on. Simple.

Take 15 minutes after you are done reading this to view yourself from a different angle. Temporary put your ego to sleep and analyze. No judgments, simply observe from afar. You'll be stunned by your findings. You'll see many silly and obvious errors you were clearly displaying. You'll wonder how you spent so many years missing these quirks.

Oh well, better late than never.

Aim to do this exercise 3 times a week for effective results.

Life HACK:

Decorate your room with posters, items, pictures of stuff that align with your long-term vision.

All these items NEED to make you feel.

Highly effective way to communicate with the subconscious.

You will now see your vision when you wake up & before you go to sleep.

How to introspect your past & present in order to clarify your future

If you don't find any flaws in yourself while introspecting, then you are not introspecting. You are simply having an ego stroking session.

What's the point of going thru a life experience if you are never going to learn from it? It's baffling how many people overlook the whole introspection process. How do I know? Because I use to be one of those people.

But introspection holds more answers than you can possibly imagine. Believe it or not, you already have most of the answers that you seek, you just haven't bought awareness to it.

Don't know what your life purpose is? Pause & take a walk down memory lane!

But be careful, make sure you are walking down memory lane correctly, or you may get hit with a truck.

Aimlessly looking in the past is dangerous. When you aimlessly look at the past, you only come out with regret. Switch your strategy.

Level Up Mentality

Purposely look at the past. And the way you do that is by looking at your past with the **sole** intention of picking up lessons that you overlooked.

If you don't have clue what to introspect on, then find use your regrets as a compass:

1. Find 1 thing from your past that you regret.

2. Find 3 lessons from that regret.

3. Apply those 3 lessons in the future.

It will feel like an anchor from your body has been removed.

The more anchors that you remove, the more clarity that you gain. And the more clarity you gain, the more you see what you eventually overlooked.

Is that your life purpose you see?

Who knows, you need to go on and give this exercise a try.

Final Thoughts about the North Star

We have the tendency to want everything to go perfect before we begin. We await the right time, approval from our peers & clear signals to start.

But want to know something?

There is never a right time. If you are awaiting the right time, then you will be waiting forever. The greatest accomplishments came to those people who began before they were ready. And that's how you need to approach your level up journey as well.

The thing about your life purpose is that it is never set in stone, it is something that evolves with time. As you accumulate new experiences, mature, meet new people, your live purpose may refine & change.

And that is completely normal. Expecting your life purpose to remain the same for your entire life robs you off growth & the potential to find something better.

But in order to refine & clarify your north star, you **need** to begin. The longer you sit on the sidelines, the more you will overthink. The more you overthink, the more you will begin to doubt yourself. Soon, you will quit the race, even before you begun.

With that being said, begin today. Your job is not to get it perfect from the get go. Your job is to start & perfect it from there.

Now experiment, carve out a path & turn your hazy north star into a clear one.

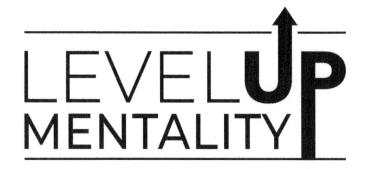

PART 4:
Controlling Your Mind

The 2 Minds

Learn to control your thoughts so you can control your behavior. Learn to control your behavior so you can control your actions. Learn to control your actions so you can control your results. Learn to control your results so you can control your legacy.

A few years ago, my friend asked me a question on how I view the mind. That question got me thinking...

What exactly is the mind? Because the brain is a physical entity. But you can't quite see the mind, it's just there. Heck, you are using the mind to read these words right now!

As I went onto research this question for many years, I came out with 1 major realization. The question was phrased incorrectly. The correct way to phrase the question should have been:

How do you view the minds?

There were 2 minds all along: The conscious & subconscious mind.

The conscious mind is your critical thinking mind & your subconscious mind is your emotional feeling mind.

Your ego, your sense of self, is the mind that rests between your conscious & subconscious mind.

So which mind has a bigger influence on your reality? It is the subconscious mind, not even close. The subconscious mind dictates at least 95% of your reality.

At the core of it, you are an emotional creature. So it should not be too much of a surprise that your emotional feeling mind has so much of a say for your current day self. A human typically feels the emotion first, then processes the information with logic.

But you need to make sure that you are aware of this concept because the emotional feeling mind will lead to a lot of irrational decisions, if you let it.

Picture a fear that you currently have. Let's say you are terrified of public speaking.

If a person who has massive speech anxiety is called on stage, they will feel terror & try to avoid it. Is this a logical choice? Not really. The person has to go on stage for 5-8 minutes, speak, get off stage, and then everyone can go back to their day.

But that's not what happens. This individual feels the fear first, finds a way to not get up on stage, THEN tries to logically explain the decision. 'Well, I was feeling sick' they say.

After reading this, you may feel guilty for pulling a similar stunt sometime in your life.

But the ultimate point is that your emotional mind is dictating a large part of your reality. And your emotional mind loves comfort. This is the main reason why so many people stay in the comfort zone. Their conscious mind may want more, but the crippling paralysis of fear is holding them back.

However, your conscious mind has the POWER to override the subconscious mind. When you are able to use your thinking mind to override the emotional mind, you have shown COURAGE.

Anytime you have done something brave in your life, I guarantee your heart was beating nonstop beforehand. But you showed the grit to continue anyways. That's how you grow as a person.

But the emotional mind is not some sort of monster that is holding you back. It is a database of your life, designed to do things to keep you safe. In many cases, it will look out for you when you aren't aware.

Ever had a gut instinct that you couldn't quite explain? Something felt off about someone, but you felt like you were being silly. So, you decided to go with your logical mind & brushed off this illogical feeling. But as you progressed on with this person, you realized that your gut was right. Sound familiar?

Well guess what, your emotional feeling mind is also responsible for the gut instinct! It thinks in terms of energy, an extremely valuable tool when dealing with humans.

The 2 minds will help guide you in your journey. But understand that you need to find a balance:

-If you think too much with your feelings & ignore your logic, then you risk acting impulsive.

-If you think too much with your logical mind & ignore your feelings, then you risk ignoring your intuition.

It was Lao Tzu who said:

'Mastering others is strength. Mastering yourself is true power.'

Finding the true balance your logical mind & emotional mind is a lifelong journey. It's not something that you will learn to operate in a book. It is something you will learn from pain, failures, wisdom & introspection.

As you grow & mature, you will feel a stronger grasp of your internal world. The stronger your grasp becomes, the more progress you begin to master yourself.

Is an Ego a Bad thing?

Too much ego = Egotistical

Too little ego = Pushover

Tamed ego = Clarity

An ego can be your best friend or your worst enemy. The ego is your sense of self, your identity. It is the mind that rests between your conscious & subconscious mind.

But unfortunately, the ego has gotten a bad reputation in the real world. However, that is highly misguided! You NEED an ego.

Why is it important? Because your ego gives you a sense of purpose. By trying to eliminate your ego, you try to eliminate your sense of self. By trying to eliminate your sense of self, you become a people pleaser whose sole goal is to live off approvals.

An ego is necessary for your level up journey. But an ego comes in two forms: untamed & tamed.

An untamed ego is when your ego rules you. This is the type of ego that you do not want.

Signs of an Untamed Ego:

Narrow minded

Reactive

Narcissistic

Interrupts others

An untamed ego will make your level up journey feel like mission impossible. You will rub a lot of people the wrong way & make a lot of short-sighted decisions. Which is why you need to tame the ego!

Taming the ego is no easy task. It often happens in the darkness. 6 ways to tame the ego are:

-Shame

-Things going wrong

-Reflection

-Added perspectives

-Meditation

Level Up Mentality

-Awareness

Taming your ego means that you no longer think everyone should live by your reality. You understand that everyone is living in their own world as well. This helps you feel more liberated because you no longer think that everyone is watching you.

Once you tame it, you leverage your ego to make constructive responses & not destructive reactions.

This transition is huge because now your ego no longer rules you. Rather, you rule it & use it as a tool.

Having a tamed ego has you fueling your ambition & striving for growth. But more importantly, your tamed ego helps you make intelligent decisions that help you in the long term.

Signs of a Tamed Ego:

Open Mind

Compassionate

Responsive

Great listener

Your ego is your sense which influences your self-esteem. So make sure you are leveraging a tamed ego to level up rather than an untamed ego to level down.

Designing an Alter Ego

Create an alter ego of the best version of yourself. Then become best friends with your alter ego. You will feel extra confident & unstoppable.

'When do I know if I have become best friends with my alter ego?

When you become your alter ego.

Around my early 20s, I went on a journey to become my best friend. I am an engineer who had built systems for multiple industries. There had to be a way for me to design a system for my life. Hmm...

I read books, watched videos, asked mentors etc. But every time I searched for the answers externally, I was left feeling disappointed. Which was why I decided to take matter into my own hands.

After a long time and a boat load of trial & errors, I came to a conclusion:

Writing & speaking was the answer!

We have a lot of thoughts & feelings flowing through us on a daily basis. If you Google how much thoughts you have throughout the day, the number is more than 30,000! So, you need to get them from your internal world onto the external world.

Step 1- Create the alter ego

Now that you have a life purpose, you need to design the alter ego to reach that purpose. Remember:

In order to get what you want, you have to act like the person who has already gotten it.

This should be an image of your best self. My recommendation is to listen to gym music and think BIG. Create the perfect being in terms of emotionally, physically, financially, spiritually etc.

Step 2. Write

Most people journal about their past or present. However, with this strategy, we are going to switch is up. Put your mindset in your alter ego's mind & give your present day self, advice. Talk about whatever. Any tough moments in your life, have your alter ego guide you out of it. Analyze your moves together. TALK LIKE FRIENDS.

Step 3. Mirror

Now do the same strategy, but in front of a mirror. Make direct eye contact & speak. Have your alter ego tell you anything relevant to help you reach your best self.

Step 4. Audio Download Audacity + buy a USB mic, or just download a recorder on your phone

Do the same thing as the prior steps but record yourself. This is your audio journal. Listen back to your talk once you are done.

'Why am I doing all of this??'

Because you are rewiring your subconscious mind. By writing & speaking everything into existence, then reading & listening back to it, you are creating & consuming the words of a new being, your alter ego.

'How long does it take for me to notice changes?'

Depends.

I've seen differing results. Took me 2-3 months of consistently doing it every day to see huge changes. The only way to find out is by executing on this strategy.

Few bonus effects of this formula:

1. You become a better writer since you are writing every day.

2. Your body language improves because you are speaking in front of the mirror every day.

3. You become a better speaker because you are recording yourself speaking everyday.

This strategy isn't something that you will find on Google. I just discovered this on my own while trying to experiment with mind rewiring tactics.

Do not think this strategy will excuse you from putting in work!

This strategy will make your conscious & subconscious mind work together so you can feel in more control over your life. But you still need to put in a lot of work for your dreams. Do not just sit on your ass writing & talking then go back to watching Worldstar all day.

Speak & consume the words of your alter ego, until one day, you become it.

Rewire Your Mentality with Awareness

Interrupting your thoughts is how you rewire your mentality.

1. *Make yourself aware when you get in a negative thought loop.*

2. *Interrupt it.*

3. *Replace it with an empowering thought.*

Each time you interrupt, each time you've completed a mental rep.

You work out your body, right?

'Yes.'

What about your mind?

'No.'

Well it's time to change that. A mental rep is no different than a bicep curl. A mental rep is strength training for the mind.

The key component of mental training is **awareness**. The more you train your awareness, the stronger your mind power becomes.

1. **Make yourself aware when you get in a negative thought loop-** Your mind is naturally inclined to think negative thoughts for survival reasons. When you understand this core concept, it's much easier to do something about it.

-Awareness = Noticing without judgment

2. **Interrupt it-** Once you have made yourself aware, you have gained a significant amount of power back. Most people don't make it to step 2 because they just let the negative thoughts play out. But you are going to interrupt! How? Through replacement.

3. **Replace with empowering thought-** Remember grasshopper, you don't stop thinking thoughts, you REPLACE thoughts. Replace the negative thought with an empowering one.

-You can try thinking it, saying it or writing it.

That's a mental rep! The more reps you do, the more you:

☆ weaken your negative neural pathways.

☆ strengthen your positive neural pathways.

Level Up Mentality

Lifechanging stuff if you consistently take your brain to the gym. The stronger the mind, the easier the life.

Rule Your Mind

Turn shame into motivation.

Turn haters into witnesses.

Turn fear into a compass.

Turn shyness into charisma.

Turn low self-worth into Godlike confidence.

Perception.

You view life the way YOU want.
You rule your mind, not the other way around.

Act like it.

Bridging the 2 Minds

Breathing is controlled by your subconscious mind.

Awareness is controlled by your conscious mind.

The more you meditate, the more you build a bridge between the 2 minds.

Stronger bridge leads to:

☆ *Added confidence*

☆ *Less anxiety*

☆ *Sharpened focus*

Meditation will allow you to unlock a new portal, don't sleep on it now. Let's begin with the WHY behind meditation. Currently, you have the monkey mind. Your mind is restless & your thoughts are uncontrolled.

Uncontrolled thoughts -> Uncontrolled emotions -> Anxiety

The reason why you are doing meditation is to tame your mind. Currently, you are your mind's bitch. You blindly follow its irrational thoughts & don't even know it. We want you to become the RULER.

'How do I do that bucko?'

By building the invisible bridge between your 2 minds. By masterfully designing this bridge, you will become the ruler of your kingdom.

There are tons of meditation tactics out there, but I will be describing the breath meditation.

How to do Breathing Meditation:

1. Find a quiet area.

2. Close your eyes.

3. Count your NATURAL breaths.

4. When you get lost in thought, make yourself AWARE, and count your breaths again.

You'll lose count of your breath many times, but don't sweat it. Meditation must be done *without* judgment. The main thing you're going for is making yourself AWARE.

EACH TIME YOU MAKE YOURSELF AWARE, THE STRONGER THE BRIDGE BECOMES.

Level Up Mentality

The awareness allows your conscious mind to make eye contact with your subconscious mind. The core principle of meditation is exercising your awareness.

The stronger your awareness muscle becomes, the more your monkey mind melts. The stronger your bridge becomes, the more you feel whole.

You feel more alive than ever.

Now you have entered a new portal. You will notice how the mass majority spend their lives running around with a monkey mind, but not you. You have tamed your mindset.

With that being said, make meditation more than an act, make it a lifestyle. Start off with 5 min a day & work your way up. Each time you meditate without skipping a day, each time you get closer to momentum.

Momentum will allow you to control your thoughts at will.

Momentum will allow you to control your emotions at will.

Momentum will allow you to control your breaths at will.

Momentum will allow you to control your reality at will.

Now go! Meditate every day for the rest of your LIFE. And discover the untapped potential of your mind.

The Difference between Meditation & Mindfulness

'What's the difference between meditation & mindfulness?'

For me, meditation is an activity & mindfulness is a lifestyle.

I set aside time to meditate like an activity. And I aim to do mindfulness throughout the day like a lifestyle. Both plays off one another.

'What do you mean both plays off one another?'

Basically, when you mediate more, you become more mindful & when you are mindful, it is easier to meditate.

Meditation is when you set aside time to bring your focus on something in the present moment like your breath, an object, physical sensations etc.

Mindfulness is when you make yourself aware throughout the day. When you catch yourself drifting into your head as you are tackling you day, make yourself aware & come back to the present.

Example: Say you are having a conversation with someone & they are telling you a story. You are dozing off & daydreaming.

Make yourself aware of your daydreaming & then come back to the present moment to pay attention.

Doing both in unison is a fantastic way to build your awareness & stay present in the moment on autopilot. Aim to do both daily.

The Mind Body Connection

Have you ever had that moment where you are feeling sad & out it, but then you fixed your posture & you didn't feel as bad?

I recommend you give it a try the next time you are feeling blue.

This phenomenon is what I call the body & mind connection:

The body influences the mind & the mind influences the body.

This is an important concept to understand because it is easier to control the body rather than the mind. We can't always control our thoughts, but we can always control our posture.

Your posture & ability to smile will impact your thoughts for the best. Slouching & frowning will impact your thoughts for the worst.

So if the body is so important, are you making the effort to take care of it? Or are you someone who is munching on fast food & drinking soda all day?

It's important that you begin making your body a priority as it is impacting your mind:

Level Up Mentality

Mind - meditate, read, watch empowering content, visualize, journal, converse with high value people.

Body - eat healthy, stay hydrated, get sun, lift weights, yoga, do cardio & play sports.

A healthy body has a spillover effect that has you improving many other facets of your life. One of the best ways to gear your life towards the right path is by enhancing your body, which will enhance your mind, which will enhance your emotions & so on.

Mind Body Challenge

Go on a 120-day body challenge.

Workout & eat right.

'Okay you just mentioned the body.'

If you are able to complete the full 120 days, then you will realize you mainly worked out your mind.

Confidence: How Values Create Value

'I want to be confident. How can I make people like me?'

Stop. Confidence is when you don't care if people like you.

'Don't care if people like me? That doesn't sound right.'

Counterintuitive, I know. But trust me, adopting this mindset will make your life 10x easier.

There are 2 forms of confidence:

1. **External-** This form of confidence is when the external world influences your self-value. When you think that Ferrari, mansion, blinged out jewelry will make all your problems go away. But this confidence comes with a catch.

'And what is that?'

This confidence is very volatile. Basing your worth off items comes with pros & cons. One pro is that it's quick. If you're making money, you can buy items & immediately feel good about yourself.

The bad part is that as you mature, you do not place as much value on items alone. You go from valuing items to people. Once the transition happens, all the items that once made you feel good, doesn't have the same effect.

Another risky thing about external confidence is that it's fickle. I mean you are buying a lot of things not only to feel good about yourself, but you want others to check out your status. This causes you to commit a social dynamics sin.

'Which is?'

Basing your value on the opinions of others. You cannot control other people's opinions, so allowing that to be your baseline for confidence comes back to bite you.

Adopting the external confidence approach may have you feeling good initially, but after some time, you'll be back to your insecure self.

2. **Internal**- This path allows you to have full control. All your powers come from within. This is self-confidence. This route takes longer but is 100% worth it.

With this route, you care about your own opinion the most & don't care if people like you. You don't try to impress anyone but yourself. This surprisingly makes people like you *more*. You embody a sense of self-assuredness that puts others at ease.

'So how do I get internal confidence?'

Few ways:

-Overcome a few insecurities.

Level Up Mentality

-Build skillsets.

-Complimenting yourself more.

-Helping others become better versions of themselves.

But there's one that is very important.

'Which is?'

Values.

'Values? What is that going to do?'

It keeps you grounded. It gives you something to stand for. And most importantly? It connects you with your internal world. By creating values for your life, you slowly transition into becoming your best friend.

But there's a catch. You need to be **firm** with your values. Anytime you break your values, you lose a grip with the internal world. Results? The conflicts of the external world will begin to rattle you more.

However, if you stick to them, your power grows & you become well grounded. The conflicts of the external world do not phase you as much. You now become your own leader in life. That's true internal confidence. You feel bold because now you are your harshest critic & biggest fan.

And just like that, you have your changed reality.

'Have you tried both strategies?'

I have. Growing up, I went the external confidence route. Did wonders in the beginning, but eventually fizzled out. For the past few years, I have been doing the internal confidence route.

'And how have you been feeling?'

Better than ever. It's definitely a process. Every day you get to know yourself on a deeper level. And the more that you learn about yourself, the more that you want to know! Life becomes so much easier because now you feel in control.

Now choose your path.

Valuing yourself is a major key to getting ahead in life. Stop treating yourself like a clearance item & begin treating yourself like a luxury product! Love yourself & you will begin to attract quality people.

Build Houses, Towers & Castles of Confidence

The reason that many people never feel confident is because they never acknowledge their accomplishments. They cross off a bunch of goals & immediately are onto the next one. This will have you always feeling unfulfilled. Slow down. ACKNOWLEDGE your accomplishments.

The secret to confidence is **gratitude**. Gratitude is acknowledging your small & big wins in life. Basically, you are bragging about yourself, to yourself.

Brick Cement Mentality: Your accomplishments are the bricks. Your acknowledgment is the cement.

Imagine stacking a bunch of bricks without any cement. Would the final product be firm & durable?

'No.'

Why?

'Because the bricks without cement creates a flimsy final product.'

Exactly.

Same with your life. Stacking up accomplishments without ever taking the time to acknowledge them will have you feeling flimsy.

'Is that why I have so much to be grateful for, yet I feel unfulfilled?'

Yes. You are a pile of bricks that is in desperate need of some cement.

But acknowledge your accomplishments & you will turn those bricks into houses, towers & castles.

'What's the best way to acknowledge my accomplishments?'

Keep it light hearted & fun. You don't need to list out your accomplishments in a robotic way. Remember, your subconscious mind is like a playful kid. So compliment yourself like you are talking to a friend. Very important!

In order to change your inner voice, you need to change your outer voice. Get in the habit of speaking empowering thoughts out loud. Do this for long enough & your inner voice will follow suit.

Do this every day from here on out. I don't care how small the accomplishment is, acknowledge it! Here's a small exercise for you get started.

Grateful Whiteboard Challenge:

1. Buy a whiteboard to hang in your room.

2. Make a list of the stuff you're grateful for. You can add onto the list as you stack up more accomplishments.

3. Read it out loud when you wake up & before you go to bed.

4. Do it forever.

Gratitude will have your life changing for the best. That is how you unlock confidence.

Mental Toughness

Mental toughness is something that you will never be taught. You must be exposed to tough experiences to give birth to a tough mind.

One of the most unique life ironies I have discovered is:

The harder life becomes, the tougher your mind becomes.

The tougher your mind becomes, the easier life becomes.

In my eyes, mental toughness is one of the biggest facets of intelligence in the real world. Without a tough mind, every challenge feels like you are hitting a wall. However, with mental toughness, every problem seems like a solution in the making.

A tough mind is very similar to going to the gym & lifting without gloves.

'What's the correlation?'

When you don't wear gloves to the gym, you'll notice you feel a strong sense of pain when the weights cause friction against your skin. The pain has you considering whether you should invest in gloves or not. But you decide to continue on.

Level Up Mentality

Session after session, you expose yourself to the weights & put up with the friction that is left on your palms. However, you show up anyways.

After a few sessions go by, you notice something. You have callus on your palms. All the friction has toughened up your palms & now you don't even notice when there is friction.

Does that mean the friction went away? No! It means your palms have toughened up & you are able to easily brush it off.

This concept is very similar to mental toughness. You ever heard the quote: Life never gets easier, you just get stronger.'

That quote is 100% true. Your challenges will never go away, but rather, your mind will simply get tougher over time. In order to unlock mental toughness, you need to expose yourself to tough events that scare you & make you second guess yourself. You need to invite friction into your life.

With each friction, you will feel dark emotions, internal pain & a strong desire to quit. Even though you want to quit, you realize that the struggles are simply a workout for your internal world. You continue forward no matter how difficult it feels & slowly begin to make gradual progress & tackle each challenge.

Just like how you didn't give up in the gym when the weights were burning you, you mustn't give up when the experiences are burning you.

Persevere no matter how hard it gets, glory awaits.

The Evolution of The Minds in the Level Up Journey

The beauty about the level up journey is that you begin to engineer your own life rather than having life be designed for you. The best way to do that is by having your subconscious mind & conscious mind working together. Apply the practical tips discussed in this section & aim to reach harmony.

When your critical thinking mind can work with your emotional feeling mind, you unlock a level of growth that hacks your life for the best.

The 2 minds will continue to evolve as you strive to make each day better. Enjoy the process but be sure to strive for more. You stop growing, when you decide to. Make growth a lifelong mantra, and your level up journey will be fun. Now let's move onto how the mind can work with another core part of you, your emotions.

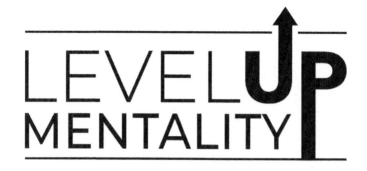

PART 5:

Working With
Your Emotions

What is Emotional Intelligence?

In my eyes, emotional intelligence is one of the most impactful subjects to immerse yourself in. During your level up journey, you will be battletested like none other. Stretching past the comfort zone comes with the good, the bad & the ugly. In order to make your journey smoother, it is imperative that you can work with your emotions rather than against them.

At the end of the day, emotions = energy in motions. It is simply energy that your body produces depending on certain circumstances.

But emotional intelligence is highly misunderstood by the general public. The main misconception is that someone who is emotionally intelligent makes emotional decisions.

Wrong.

It's the exact opposite.

Someone who is emotionally intelligent can acknowledge their emotions without judgment, aim to understand what the emotions are trying to tell them, then make a RATIONAL decision.

The problem with a lot of society is that they lack emotional intelligence. And when you lack emotional intelligence, you get impulsivity.

Pretty sure you went thru impulsive moments in your life. Let me present to you 2 different scenarios:

Scenario A:

A car cuts you off, you feel angry, then you go into road rage mode. You begin to tailgate the car, flick them off, and go on a journey to cut them off as well. Your behavior opens you up to getting a ticket, getting in a car accident, or worse, losing your life. Was that a rational decision? Absolutely not. And the reasons that you behaved like this was because you allowed your emotions to rule you.

Scenario B:

Someone cuts you off in traffic, you feel angry, but you decide that road rage will not solve anything. So you hold that anger, drive over to the gym, and lift weights like a warrior. In this case, you have leveraged your emotions for growth. You responded to the situation & made a rational decision.

In many ways, emotional intelligence will make you mature faster. Think about it, what is maturation? In my eyes it is the ability to respond rather than react. Picture the most mature person that you know. Do you think that they don't fell strong, disruptive, dark emotions at times? Of course, they do! But they do not let those emotions control them.

Immature: Emotions overpower the mind.

Mature: Mind overpowers the emotions.

In order to be emotionally intelligent, you need to master one major facet of your life: your breath.

A quiet, slow breath equals a happy life. Give this a try:

NINJA BREATHS:

Breathe in & out thru your nose.

Should be silent.

If you hear noise, you are doing it wrong.

You will silence your breath by slowing down.

Once 'silent mode' is activated, you have achieved deep breathing. Diaphragm is now engaged.

Shallow breaths no more.

Each time you have corrected your breath, you have tamed your emotions. That's an internal rep. You have harmonized your mind & emotions. Wow look at you! You are becoming emotionally intelligent before my eyes.

Now keep going.

Becoming your Own Best Friend

Becoming best friends with yourself happens in the darkness. When you hit rock bottom, you have nowhere else to go. That's when you MUST get to know all of yourself. The good & ESPECIALLY the bad. Once that happens, you now have your back for life, best friend status.

'Does it have to be in the darkness? Why can't I become best friends with myself in the light?'

Because you're missing one key element.

'Which is?'

Friction.

Friction is what allows you to see if a friendship is legit or fake.

Friction moves past words alone & sheds light into the actions.

Everyone can be there for you when things are fine and dandy. At that point, they have their words to fall back on. Which is why the comfort zone will have you feeling more popular than ever.

126

Level Up Mentality

But in the darkness? Things begin to change. This is the stage where action takes over. At this point, a lot of 'friends' start disappearing & only a few will remain.

Now having friends from the external world who stick by your side is great. But you must take it a level further.

'How?'

You need to go internal.

Even the world's greatest empath will NEVER be able to fully feel your pain. Only YOU will be able to feel that. Whether it's the death of a loved one, a car accident, going broke etc. You need to begin this journey.

'What journey?'

The journey to make sense of the pain.

'Is it okay if I feel scared?'

Yes & most people do. In fact, they feel so scared, that they do everything in their power to avoid this journey. They turn to alcohol, drugs, excessive partying etc. Anything that they can think of to run away from beginning.

But the rare few? They begin. Despite feeling some nerves, they enter the unknown.

-They learn about their pain.

-They make sense of their inner demons.

-They battle darkness day in & day out like a fucking warrior.

Each day as they move forward in this path, each day they learn more about themselves. Day by day, the unknown is becoming clearer. And the clearer the unknown becomes, the stronger the bond with your internal world grows.

Soon enough, you begin to understand yourself on a deeper level. You have always known the good sides to you, but now? You also know the bad sides.

And when you officially understand the good AND the bad, you have survived the journey. You now have your back for LIFE. You feel more confident than EVER.

'Really??'

Yes.

☆ Confidence = Best friends with yourself.

So if you are going thru a dark time right now, understand the only way to overcome it is by entering the unknown & making sense of the pain.

Keep pushing forward& chronicle your journey out of the abyss. Then look back with pride once you overcame the adventure that many were afraid to take.

Your best friend waits on the other end.

Why Being Scared is a Good Thing

The more you fail, the less you fear it.

The less your fear it, the more you grow.

The more you grow, the less you settle.

The less you settle, the more you build.

✰ More building = More Creation = Your Masterpieces = Your Legacy

Fear makes you human. No one wants to fail & make a fool of themselves. This is why many people choose to settle in life.

There are 2 kinds of fear:

Fear 1 (Threat) - this is a legitimate fear that can put your safety at risk.

Fear 2 (Illusion of Threat) - a false fear that is not rational created by limiting beliefs.

Confusing fear 2 as fear 1 is why many people never leave their comfort zone.

This is the reason why exiting the comfort zone is so difficult. It's because you are battling a lot of dark emotions to venture past it when you level up. But this is a good sign on your end!

When you feel scared & do something anyways, that shows courage. If you don't ever feel scared, then you should be alarmed. Chances are that you are not challenging yourself.

Courage isn't the absence of fear. It is continuing despite feeling fear. Get it? It is okay to be nervous before you are about to be brave.

Don't be ashamed of fear. From here on out, use it as a form of encouragement. Understand that this emotion is serving as your compass in the level up journey. Once you begin welcoming failures into your life, you will notice something magical happen.

You will notice that the emotions that once crippled you are now the same emotions that fuel you and make you feel alive. Once that transition occurs, you can confidently acknowledge that you have reconditioned your perception towards failure.

That's when things get fun.

Jealousy Gets a Bad Reputation

You ever had that moment when you feel a strong surge of jealousy & become highly alert?

Maybe one of your close friends bought a new Mercedes & made you aware of it. You felt jealousy & wondered, why him & not me? What makes him so special to earn this beautiful Mercedes, while I am driving my mom's old Buick?

Nothing against Buick's by the way.

You my friend, are jealous. Is that a bad thing? Well, depends.

Jealousy in itself is not a bad thing to experience. It is a primal emotion. But your reaction to jealousy will determine whether you are a winner or a loser.

Loser: Use jealousy to admit defeat & become a hater or a snake in the process.

Winner: Use jealousy to become inspired & use it as a compass on which goal to tackle next.

In the level up world, we adopt the life of a winner, which is why jealousy is a good thing. Jealousy creates internal motivation & an internal compass. If something is making you jealous, then there is a great opportunity for you to introspect.

Sometimes, the trigger that sparked your jealousy was blown way out of proportion, so you can brush it off. But other times, the trigger that sparked your jealousy requires further looking into to. Jealousy gives you a peak into your hidden desires & allows you to see what you crave.

Why not make a goal out it? If you want it bad enough & another human is able to obtain that goal, then so can you!

And to be honest, if you hang with a bunch of winners, then you will find yourself getting jealous very often. But use that jealousy as inspiration to take your game up another notch. Results? Chain effect of more winning.

Every emotion serves a bigger picture in the grand scheme of things. Make sure you are leveraging your internal energy & not wasting it on finger pointing.

Now level up.

Dealing with Embarrassment

A part of growth is willing to embarrass yourself. But want to know something? Embarrassment is a learned act. You rarely got embarrassed as a little kid. You didn't give a fuck. But as you grew older, the self-consciousness kicked it. It's time to strip that away by unlocking your inner child.

'How do I unlock my inner child?'

Good question. There are plenty of ways to go about it. But I'm going to give you my formula.

Unlock Your Inner Child Formula:

1. Make fun of yourself when you fail.

2. Smile more.

3. Talk to other people's inner child.

1. Make fun of yourself when you fail.

When you were a kid, you didn't view it as failing. You viewed it as trying. Nowadays, you get all mopey when you take a loss. Fix that. Aim to roast yourself when you fail at something. This HACK reconditions your perception towards losses.

2. Smile more.

Smiling releases endorphins in your brain. Endorphins are feel good chemicals. Which is why you need to smile more. Heck, hold a smile for 2-3 minutes soon as you wake up. Notice your day go 10x better. Magic.

3. Talk to other people's inner child.

☆Talking to someone's adult side builds an acquaintance.

☆Talking to someone's child side builds a friend.

A human's inner child never goes away, it just gets buried due to life's responsibilities. Talk to them like they were 5 years old.

Bonus Tip: Read the books that you read as a kid, preferably fiction. This helps your brain disrupt the logical patterns it has been conditioned with. You begin to think more freely.

Do these steps & the inner child in you will awaken once more. You know, the free spirit that didn't give a fuck about opinions? The only thing they gave a fuck about were their curiosities & how they could have fun.

Get it?

☆Curiosity + Fun = CHEATCODE for Growth

You need your spirits by your side if you want to level up.

While most people are being mopey & being self-conscious to try new things, you do the exact opposite. You hacked your life & brought out what society tried to suppress, **your imagination.**

When you control your imagination, you control your reality. No longer will you use your imagination to pre plan your failures. But now? You will use it to pre plan your rise. Gamechanger.

Life changes when you are ready to quit settling. Give this unorthodox life hack a try. You'll see yourself grow & have fun at the same damn time!

Mind HACK: Reframing Embarrassment

View all embarrassing moments as 'funny stories in the making. This does 2 things:

1. Forces your mind to think long term.

2. Brings humor into the mix.

A combination of the 2 is deadly & will skyrocket your growth.

Bonus: You become a better storyteller.

The Truth Behind Anxiety

Fantasy: worrying about tomorrow, will bring you peace for tomorrow.

Reality: worrying about tomorrow, will take away your peace from today.

During my college days, I had massive speech anxiety. Before giving a speech, my body would begin malfunctioning. I would get a rapid heartbeat, excessive thoughts of failing, sweaty palms and all that.

And as my body began to flood with these sensations, I began to do my best to suppress the emotions so I could deliver the speech with poise. But the more I tried to suppress the emotions, the worst that it got. And as the feelings were getting worse, I felt like giving a speech was a bad idea. I would then give the speech with a quivering voice, darting eyes, & a lack of composure.

5 years later, times are different. Nowadays, I am giving speeches in keynote events, weddings, Toastmasters competitions to audiences that go up to 350+ people. But the weird thing? I am actually excited about it! So what changed?

My tactic.

Younger me would try to suppress anxiety. My present day self embraces anxiety.

Making this mentality shift will allow you to change your perception towards anxiety. This is a life changing concept, so pay attention.

A core principle in the emotional intelligence world is:

An emotion that is attempted to be buried will go to the gym & come back 10x stronger.

Which is why suppressing a negative emotion is a misguided strategy. Not only are you making the emotion worse, but you are conditioning a negative perception towards the emotion.

You should not be suppressing, but rather making yourself **aware**.

When you make yourself aware of a negative emotion, you simply observe without judgment. You feel the rapid heartbeat, sweaty palms & observe the negative thought from afar. When you observe emotions from afar, you make a surreal observation:

-Emotions are not the boogeyman. Emotions are simply physical sensations with a perception attached to it.

When you make this observation, you are able to CHOOSE the perception that you want to assign to an emotion.

When I realized that my emotions before a speech would never go away, I decided to embrace the feelings rather than run away from it. When I did that, I realized the emotions were not that bad.

And when my conscious mind was able to understand the subconscious feeling without judgment, I was able to view:

Anxiety -> Excitement.

If you think about it, anxiety & excitement are the same exact feelings. You feel the same way before a roller coaster as you do before a speech. But one excites you & the other terrifies you. See the problem with that?

Anxiety is simply a manmade word that forces a negative perception. Take back control of your life. Because believe me, you will be feeling a boat load of 'anxiety' in the level up journey. But from here on out, it is excitement.

That is the truth about anxiety, my friend. This emotion was never your enemy. It was simply energy that your body was providing you to knock your goals out of the park.

Time to recondition your perception towards anxiety & become best friends with it.

Let's get it.

The Emotional Pain of Loneliness

Loneliness makes you trust too quickly. You want to open up & talk to someone. But this can have you saying too much to the wrong people. Quiet. Let the trust build on its natural pace, no need to rush.

'Is being alone & lonely the same thing?'

Not quite. Alone is a physical state, lonely is a mental state.

There are a lot of people who are alone, but do not feel lonely. And there are a lot of people who are surrounded by people but feel lonely.

People feel lonely for 2 main reasons:

-They think no one cares about them.

-They have the wrong friends.

-**They think no one cares about them:** This group tends to chill by themselves a lot. During their time alone, they create mental scenes as to why more people don't hit them up. They crave more social interactions.

-They have the wrong friends: This group is rarely found by themselves. Being by themselves scare them. So, they always surround themselves with people to avoid their inner voice.

Whichever category that you fall in, understand one thing. Your bond with your internal world is weak. And when your bond with your internal world is weak, you look to the external world for answers.

Instead of fixing the relationship that you have with yourself, you think other people are going to solve it. Which is why you trust so quickly! You rush things hoping that the magical person will come by & make your loneliness melt.

I'm here to tell you that won't work. Because if you aren't happy by yourself, you will never be happy around others.

You need to recondition your perception towards loneliness. Understand that everyone felt lonely at one stage or another. And to be honest, you may often feel it while you are leveling up.

Why? Because many people will not opt into this level up journey like you have. Therefore, loneliness is a rite of passage towards confidence.

Remember:

☆Confidence = Being best friends with yourself.

So from here on out:

☆Loneliness = Pre-Confidence

Use this time to get to know yourself on a deeper level:

-journal

-follow your curiosities

-pick up a skill

Main goal is to be comfortable by yourself.

The more comfortable you become with yourself, the more your bond with your internal world grows. You are creating & discovering yourself. The more this happens, the more your happiness rises.

As you keep doing this, your perception towards loneliness will change because you are becoming best friends with yourself. You'll never have to worry if you are cared for. Why? Because now you care for yourself.

Once this happens, you will begin sending off the right energy to the world & attracting the right people into your life. You will no longer be giving out trust to the wrong people hoping someone gives you their time. You are much more patient.

Remember, loneliness will not just magically go away. You need to adopt an active approach & take care of business. So get up, be productive & strengthen the bond with your internal world.

Anger = Your Body's Red Bull

During high school, my parents had enrolled me into Karate. I remember I had no desire to learn Tae Kwon Do & would drag my feet before every single meeting. Why the heck would I want to go jumping around kicking bags, sparring & learning a whole bunch of other nonsense while I could be playing Jak & Daxter on my PS2?

But my parents had already paid for the classes, so I had to show up. Meeting after meeting, I showed up & gave a half assed effort. I would be there physically, but not mentally.

Well, my karate instructor had taken notice. Every few weeks, we would be given a stripe on our belt. The stripes allowed us to progress closer to the next belt.

I remember one day after an intense karate session, my instructor had given my brother his stripes, but not me. Hm, why was that? We started our karate journey on the same exact same day!

So I confronted my karate teach after the meeting, and asked him what was up. He looked at me dead in the eyes & said that I didn't deserve it. He said I was lazy, and not a hard worker like my brother. Unless I fixed my act, I would NOT be given a stripe.

This had me heated. Who the fuck was this dude to tell me that I wasn't a hard worker? His comments stung my soul but had awakened a hidden beast. I became angry & was ready to prove him wrong.

The next few sessions, I worked like a mad man & gave it a 110% effort. That effort allowed me to not only be given the stripes, but allowed me to learn an important life lesson.

Anger is your body's Red Bull.

It is the energizer drink that will have you performing at god like levels. Anger is energy that brings you alertness & allows you to 10x yourself.

If this emotion is so powerful, then why is viewed so negatively? Because most humans waste their anger on a hissy fit. Imagine if I had began whimpering like a little bitch after my karate instructor had demanded more out of me. I would have never gone on to become a black belt. I owe so much to that instructor that it is hard to put my appreciation into words.

How often have you let your anger destruct you rather than fuel you? Rather than channeling your anger into producing, you opt to let it be an excuse to destruct.

But when you use your anger to destruct, all you end up doing is feeling shame afterwards. I'm sure you have never felt proud after a temper tantrum. You simply thought 'wow, what have I done?'

Emotions are temporary. They come & go. Making impulsive decisions based off your emotions is silly. The consequences can come & stay.

Your emotions come in waves, they are not the sea. Your anger will come, and your anger will go. Don't make decisions that you regret.

TREAT ANGER LIKE YOUR BODY'S RED BULL.

It is all energy. From here on out, when you are angry, take a few controlled breaths & feel the emotion. Anger makes you stronger, more creative & more energized.

Have an outlet whenever you are angry to release the energy on. Don't bottle it up because it is destructive and can enforce a negative perception towards the emotion.

Anger is your best friend, quit treating it like an enemy.

Now use the anger & get your wings.

Humor = Modern Day Superpower

Have you ever seen a baby laugh? Pretty endearing thing to witness, right? Such a subtle act that brings joy to your heart.

You wonder what exactly made this baby burst into laughter. Was it something that you did, or did the baby have a certain thought running in their mind that made them laugh?

Whatever the case is, we are programmed to FEEL good from seeing others laugh & laughing for yourself. Laughing or making someone laugh is a modern-day superpower.

Look around you. How many people do you see with a scrunched-up sourpuss looking face? Plenty.

But these people are robbing themselves of a major life hack: **Endorphins.**

Endorphins are feel good chemicals that your brain releases which enhance your mood. But the magic is that when you laugh, you release the mirror neurons in others who end up feeling good as well.

Side Effects of Laughing:

You feel good

Level Up Mentality

You make others feel good

You enhance your likeability

You can turn a negative situation into a positive one

These are only a few effects. You need to leverage this human emotion in your level up journey.

When life is kicking your ass, the last thing you may want to do is laugh, I get it. But force yourself to do it anyways! Unleash your inner child & have a good chuckle. Guarantee it will have the power to change up your mindset & mood.

Bingo.

Ambition

It takes introspection to discover your true self. It takes ambition to discover your best self.

Top tier ambition is born thru pain. In order to run towards your grandest self, you must also be running away from something. You're running away from mediocrity, past trauma & self-doubt. When you run away fast, you move forward quicker.

What? You thought I was going to say that ambition is simply born thru wanting a good future? It is for a lot of people, sure. But *top tier* ambition requires pain. Humans are more motivated by avoiding pain rather than seeking pleasure.

But there is an art to ambition. There is an art to wanting more out of life & being happy with what you already have. This is a grateful person who is driven. A rare breed of human who enjoys the process but does not lose sight of the bigger picture.

Look around you & find the top performers in any field. You'll notice from their eyes that they have been thru a boat load of struggle to get to where they are today. Don't believe me? Then listen to some of their interviews.

The only thing that will fuel your level up journey is having the ambition to push yourself to new heights. Average bums often set a goal, reach a goal, give themselves a pat on the back & go back to watching TV.

However, someone in the level up world, sets a goal, reaches a goal, give themselves a pat on the back & goes on to find the next goal.

Ambition breeds confidence. The more that stretch past the limiting beliefs that were once placed upon you, the more that you will notice you feel more powerful in the process.

Does ambitious require work? Absolutely.

Is the work worth it? Absolutely.

Runaway from something. Run towards something. Use this formula to continue to shatter your prior day milestones.

Closing Thoughts on Emotions

Whether you view the emotion to be good or bad, just aim to keep one major concept in mind. Your emotions are energy that communicate with you.

Rather being in a rush to run away from dark emotions, run towards them. See what your internal world is trying to tell you. Typically your emotions have the answer that you are searching from in a blog, podcast or blog. Don't be in such a rush to suppress, them.

All emotions can be leveraged for growth. It may not seem like it now, but it will one day when you incorporate emotional intelligence into your life.

You will never fully understand your emotions. Rather you will continuously learn more about them as you progress in your level up journey. Good emotions will make you feel good. Dark emotions will teach you. Soon, you'll see how your internal energy helps you paint on the canvas of life. Utilize them to the best of your abilities for growth in your level up journey.

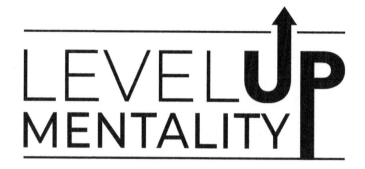

PART 6:

How to Learn & Build Skills

Level Up Lifecycle:

1. Consume.

2. Produce.

3. Teach someone how to produce.

Consumer -> Producer

Every quality producer was once a consumer who consumed with purpose.

In the real world, the energy that you put out today will one day boomerang to you. Decisions are not isolated acts, they form a chain. The question is, what kind of chain are you forming? A constructive or destructive one?

In the level up world, one mighty chain is the consumer to producer lifestyle. It is a beauty to witness because it turns you from a newbie -> competent -> master. But how is this cycle achieved? Let's break down both steps:

Consuming is when you are absorbing knowledge.

Producing is when you are applying and creating with your knowledge.

Far too often, learning is confused with action. Nope!

1. Learning = Consuming

2. Action = Producing

Both stages are needed for growth. But make sure you are not getting stuck in step 1 & confusing it as step 2. When you mistake step 1 for step 2, you get *analysis paralysis*.

I'm sure you had analysis paralysis many times in your life. You studied & studied away to a point where you were overwhelmed with information. And when your mind becomes overloaded with information, you stall out & spend too much time overthinking.

Which is why it is crucial that you consume with **purpose**.

Your main goal of consuming is to learn enough to produce. Learning is very important because it allows you to have a solid grasp on where to begin. I will cover the concepts of how to effectively learn later in this section. Once you have learned, your goal is to begin applying.

Applying allows you to learn the theory better than you learn the theory by studying it. The goal is to produce results. No need to rush it, but make sure you are getting better with each session.

After a while of applying the theory that you have learned, you will begin to solidify your neural pathways towards the act. Solidified neural pathways will lead a learned act -> habit -> **instinct**.

But remember this, becoming a producer does not mean that you stop being a consumer. A top tier producer is always learning & skyrocketing their knowledge. Be a lifelong student. As you are chasing your north star, you are going to have to leverage both, consumption & production.

If you can pair lifelong learning with the ambition to produce & apply, you become deadly in the level up world.

Spark the chain & you'll find it difficult to stop.

The Power of Curiosity

Life Irony: A dumb person pretends to be smarter than they are. A smart person pretends to be dumber than they are. The dumb person is unaware of their behavior. The smart person is perfectly aware.

This is a life irony that will clarify your understanding of curiosity. It all begins with:

Stupid people think they know everything.

Smart people think they have yet to know anything.

-One group thinks knowledge is finite.

-One group knows knowledge is infinite.

A stupid person wholeheartedly thinks that they know everything. Not due to maliciousness, but due to blindness.

Few examples of a stupid person:

-Someone who thinks education stops after school.

-Someone who shuts down any opposing viewpoints.

-A 'know it all.'

The reason they remain stupid is because they lack any ounce of humility. It requires a humble attitude to know that you will never fully know everything.

'Never??'

Never. Way too much knowledge out there.

But this is good.

'It's good that I will never know everything?'

Absolutely.

'Why?'

Because it allows you to grow for your entire life.

Picture this: *Knowledge is a ceiling.*

A stupid person who thinks they have learned it all caps out their ceiling. This results in them becoming content & ruling off further growth.

A smart person who knows they can always learn more, stretches out their ceiling. This results in ambition.

A smart person pretends to be dumber than they are because it's the ULTIMATE life hack. By telling their brain that they are not even close to knowing everything, their brain works on OVERDRIVE to learn everything.

Level Up Mentality

This is how you trick your brain into growth mode.

This is how you learn at a surreal pace.

This is how you unleash your DESIRE.

While the stupid person thinks they have the world figured out, the smart person is trying to figure out the world.

There's nothing more deadly than a human brain paired with humility. It allows you to seek answers while others sit on their ass. And the more questions you successfully answer, the clearer your mind becomes. You are in the process of unlocking your 3rd eye.

Now let me ask you, do you know everything?

'Not even close.'

So what will you do?

'I will seek the answers.'

For how long?

'For life.'

Excellent.

Let the loudmouths be loud. Their journey is already over, yours is just beginning.

The Difference Between Knowledge & Wisdom

Lessons learned the hard way are lessons learned for life. Mixing a lesson with a dark emotion makes it stickier. View it as short-term pain for a long-term reward.

Knowledge & wisdom are like cousins, they are similar, but not the same. In plain terms, knowledge is a painless process & wisdom is a painful process. You need both in your arsenal to maximize one another.

In today's information age, it is easier than ever to get knowledge. Knowledge will come from your external world. You can simply hop onto the internet and research topics that spark your curiosity & learn about it.

Wisdom, however, comes from the internal world. You need to go thru experiences in order to gain wisdom. It is often a painful process because wisdom is born thru darkness like failures, regrets & betrayal. As you are going thru many of your life experiences, it will feel like hell. But fear not, because there is a light at the end of the tunnel. ***Healed pain gives you wisdom.***

In the level up journey, as you are learning, you need to make sure you gain knowledge & apply it. Once you apply it, you will begin gaining experiences and failing. By failing, you learn lessons that will lead to wins. Those lessons will serve as the wisdom that you can apply to other facets of your life.

What's unique about life is that the more experiences that you stack up, the more you form a web. You see how lessons from one facet of your life can be applied to other facets. For example: going thru a bad breakup will provide lessons that can make you a better friend. You learn a lot about social etiquette from a failed relationship. Who would of thought, huh?

Ultimately, your losses may not make sense now, but it ultimately will. Just show the guts to apply your knowledge, take your losses like a warrior, analyze & wait for all the dots to connect.

It's all a process.

Process >> Results Lifestyle

'Why do we care more about the results than the process?'

Think about it for a second. Growing up, were you rewarded for studying or your test score?

'Test score.'

Exactly. You've been conditioned to value the results over the process for your entire life.

'But aren't the results more important than the process?'

Not quite. Both are needed for long term success. Otherwise, you will end up shooting yourself in the foot.

When you focus more on the results than the process, you start a toxic cycle. You create unrealistic expectations. Unrealistic expectations lead to rushing. Rushing leads to sloppy results.

'Any examples?'

Yep, public speaking. During my time at Toastmasters, many of my mentees wanted to become the perfect speaker overnight. They started off their journey with unrealistic expectations.

Level Up Mentality

They would come to each meeting, give a speech & get frustrated when they were not winning the Best Speaker ribbon. They had barely given 3 speeches & were already rushing the process! Results? Their mentality was thrown off. And when your mentality is thrown off, sloppy results are imminent.

Each of those kids eventually began getting frustrated rather than focusing on their improvements. Needless to say, they did not finish the Toastmasters program because they couldn't take it speech by speech.

In school, results are rewarded over the process. But in the real world, you NEED to alter your approach. Here's how:

1. **Identify your desired results**- This will require visualization. Take the time to spend visualizing what your ideal self will look, feel, think like when you reach your results. This will serve as your north star.

2. **Eyes on the present**- Now you know what you're working towards. At this point, I want you to give 110% on the present-day process. Your only focus is on steps 1-7 from below:

1. Learn

2. Do

3. Fail

4. Gather data

5. Fix weak spots & amplify strengths

6. Practice

7. Keep going thru 4-6 until learned

8. ~~Create systems~~

9. ~~Teach others~~

10. ~~Mastered~~

3. **Mentality Shift**. The mentality you had before was:

'I have so much left to go!' -Too self-defeating.

But now? Your mentality will be:

'Wow look how far I have come!' -Empowering as fuck.

Making the mentality shift is difficult. For me to make the shift, I practice these daily:

-Gratitude

-Journal my progress

These 2 tactics helped me rewire my mentality. If you can consistently apply these tips, then your mind will alter. You will realize that if you remain present and go all in on the process, then the results WILL come. Guaranteed.

Once the results come & you are getting better, time to take it up another notch! 'Which is??'

Numbers 8-10 from the list.

1. ~~Learn~~

2. ~~Do~~

3. ~~Fail~~

4. ~~Gather data~~

5. ~~Fix weak spots & amplify strengths~~

6. ~~Practice~~

7. ~~Keep going thru 4-6 until learned~~

8. Create systems

9. Teach others

10. Mastered

Once you can teach others, you will learn much more in the process. Plus, you will help someone else focus on the process over the results because you were able to change your mind set for yourself.

Learning leads to empowerment & teaching leads to fulfillment. Do both in your journey & skyrocket your growth in the process.

How to Learn Part 1: The Core

Before learning something new, watch at least 5 videos or read 5 articles about the subject. You'll notice a pattern with a few concepts repeatedly being discussed. These are the core concepts of the subject. Focus on the core & build up from there.

'Can you explain why you do this hack? Why not just dive right into the content?'

Great question. Let me give you a little insight into why I do this strategy. First let's begin with what the core concepts are.

The core concepts are the ***fundamentals***. All other concepts stem from the core. Let me ask you a question. Did you learn long division first or basic division?

'Basic.'

Why?

'Because I needed to know the fundamentals before leveling up.'

Exactly.

Nowadays, most people do the opposite. They go straight for the overarching stuff. But that only confuses you! You begin to think everything is important.

Result? *Analysis paralysis: Study Edition*

So, what should you do?

Get a few independent resources & analyze what each of them are focusing on. I like to do 5 different YouTube videos or articles about the subject. If the independent sources are all bringing up similar points, then those points are the core of a subject. Learn everything about the core & your entire learning process will become 1000x easier.

Want to know something funny? When you know the subject very well, you are going to realize the core was the most important part all along. You'll solidify the importance of the core when you are teaching another student.

Now pick a topic that relates to your north star & follow the 5 independent resources strategy. Scope thru the fluff & find out what's important.

Time is scarce, so we don't want to waste it in level up world.

Study Hack

Try this.

Whenever you are studying, pretend like you have to teach someone the content right after.

This mentality shift is huge.

You will scope thru the fluff.

And you will start paying attention only to the important points.

Level up your learning.

How to Learn Part 2: Getting your Emotions Involved

The biggest cheat code to learning something is by making it fun.

Major psychological hack. Making something fun sparks your internal desire. The internal desire is crucial to connect your brain & heart. That level of synergy will have you learning like a superstar.

The majority only learns with their head. And who can blame them? That's how we were taught in school. We were given tons of material to learn just so we could pass a test. We have been conditioned to learn only with our head. Which is why learning feels like work!

It feels like work because we are being told to consume material that we do not give a shit about. Which leads to people procrastinating, cramming & just half assing the process. Many will be able to pass the exams with the 50/50 effort, sure. But is any of the material retained? Nope. The reason it is not retained is because you are missing a key component of learning.

Desire.

'And how do I get that?'

Emotion.

You cannot only learn with your brain. You need your heart as well.

'How?'

Good question.

You can get your heart involved in many ways. I traditionally do 2 things:

1. Future projection.

2. Game.

These are my strategies, but you can experiment with your own. Heck, you may already be doing these without even knowing it!

1. **Future Projection** - I envision my future self being a pro in whatever I am trying to learn. When I was a master's student for business intelligence & systems engineering, I had to deal with certain topics that were dry.

When I was met with something dry, I envision it in my future.

'Example?'

Learning PowerShell. Scripting is cool & all, but not fun for me. So how do I make it fun? I picture myself as a future CEO who knows scripting inside & out. Knowing how to script has me automating like a star & blowing the other CEOs out of the water!

By envisioning how automating with PowerShell scripts gives me a competitive advantage, I am able to spark my desire towards the subject.

Point is, you need to get creative. Keep searching for new angles that you can apply to your subject & then make it relate to you. This sparks the desire within.

2. **Game** - I turn learning into a game. When I was learning public speaking, I had massive speech anxiety. Getting on stage was very difficult for me. So what did I do? I turned it into a game! This requires creativity to brainstorm different game tactics.

My idea of turning it into a game was by breaking it into levels. Each speech would help me reach a new level. Competing in speech competitions was like fighting a boss in a video game. Recruiting members for Toastmasters & helping them overcome their fear were cheat codes etc.

Both these strategies make you forget that you are learning. Rather, you are simply doing something because it is fun. And who doesn't want to have fun?

crickets

Exactly. You level up your learning by bringing out your inner child. That's the hidden key! Once you have your brain absorbing the content & your heart fueling the engine, you become UNSTOPPABLE.

Level Up Mentality

You are going to be learning.

You are going to be applying.

You are going to be retaining.

Congratulations, welcome to the top 3%.

Build Skills to Shatter Negative Self Talk

'Why do I have so much negative self-talk?'

Because you sit idle too much, thinking. Our brains are naturally predisposition to focus on the negatives for survival reasons. But you can change that by getting out of your head & working towards something. Action is king.

Action will also lead you to changing your thoughts.

You ever heard the term:

-Practice until you can do it.

'Yea...'

That's wrong. It's actually:

-Practice until you become it.

'Become what I practice?'

Yep! If you think about it, driving is an example. Driving is a part of your existence at this point. You can drive without thinking like you can breathe without thinking.

Your neural pathways for driving have strengthened & it gets stronger each time you get behind the wheel. And this is the exact reason why action is so important! You change your way of existence.

Skill Building = Confidence Building

Anytime you build a skill, you have structured new neural pathways. Neural pathways are a huge factor for your thoughts as well. You know how your mind defaults to negative thoughts & emotions now? That changes when you add a skill.

A lot of your thoughts will default to your new skill. I had a friend who used to be extremely negative. But then he got into Shopify, worked on the skill of sales & soon became a pro.

Nowadays, he sees sales opportunities everywhere! His brain transformed from defaulting to negative thoughts to thoughts about sales. Why? Because he added in new neural pathways which led to new thoughts.

Bottom line: You need to get your ass moving & find something to lock into. It can be a new business, public speaking, learning to sing etc. And keep practicing it until you become it!

Soon, the negative self-talk & negative emotions will take a back seat & your life will change to fuel your new skill.

Invest at least 3-6 months to a goal, or don't even bother.

The first few weeks feels like a drag. And it seems frustrating because this when you are the **most** motivated. But you need to push thru it.

'How long should I practice?'

Until the conscious becomes subconscious.

'Is the bridge between a conscious act & a subconscious act, practice?'

Correct.

The main reason humans do not see the fruits of their labor is because they do not practice long enough. You see, many have a problem with rushing. They want to pick up a new skillset, but don't want to put in the proper work. The reason they don't put in the proper work is because they aren't quite sure how to learn.

Learning a skillset is a 4-part process.

Stages of Learning:

1. Unconscious Incompetence

2. Conscious Incompetence

3. Conscious Competence

4. Unconscious Competence

The reason people quit so soon is because they try to skip steps in the stages of learning. But patience! Go thru the process in ORDER & your time will come.

Let's go thru the 4 levels of practice to make a thinking act an autopilot one.

Level 1

Unconscious Incompetence – At this stage, you are completely unaware. You are messing up nonstop, but you don't even know where. You can't tell the difference between doing it correctly & incorrectly.

Level 2

Conscious Incompetence- You continue to practice & now you're starting to see some patterns. You are still messing up a lot, but at least you can spot out where. You are now aware of the task at hand.

Level 3

Conscious Competence- After identifying the patterns & fixing it, you continue to practice some more. At this stage, you can do the task! However, there is a catch. You have to think A LOT.

You start wondering if this is how the entire process is going to be. You begin wondering if you are always going to have to think so much when executing. But don't give up yet, there is still one more level.

Level 4

Unconscious Competence- After showing grit & perseverance, you have finally reached level 4. You are now able to do the task on autopilot. You have solidified neural pathways for the task & it is now a part of your existence.

By going thru the entire stages of learning you can turn a learned act into an instinct. In your level up journey, you need to learn skill/s to reach your north star, so effective practicing is a must.

Now you know how to practice like a champ. Find the skillset that you want to master & take care of business!

Any goal will be extremely difficult before it is extremely easy. Get it? You can pretty much learn anything. You just need to show work ethic, consistency & perseverance. Do that & the world is yours.

Cheat Code to Productivity

Trick your mind.

Currently, you're looking for more ways to be productive.

Flip it.

Look for fewer ways to be distracted.

Eliminate distractions so productivity is your only option.

My recommendation is having a spot solely dedicated to getting work done.

Leverage Obsession
to Learn Skills

People hate on obsession. But obsession gets the job done faster. 2 months of Godlike focus beats 2 years of dipping your toes in it. Have obsession. Just know what to channel it on.

'If obsession is so beneficial, why does it get a bad rep?'

It gets a bad rep because it is misconstrued. The general public view obsessed people as zombies who take things too far. And granted, there are many obsessed people like that.

But there are many people who are not zombies, they are top performers. Let me explain the difference between the 2 groups & help you learn how to leverage obsession to learn at unprecedented levels.

Group 1: Zombies

They are USED by obsession. They are so possessed, that they let other parts of their life go to hell. Many are top performers, sure. But are they happy? Nope. All they do is obsessively work all day.

'Do they ever realize that they are zombies?'

Some do. Their loved ones snap them out of zombie mode by getting them to live a life. Or, they have an epiphany on their own. But the rest? They realize the error in their ways on their deathbed.

Group 2: High Performers

They USE obsession. They know that obsession is Focus's older brother. So, they know how to strategically be obsessed in their craft, without letting their life become a wreck.

When this group works, they WORK.

-They scoff at multitasking.

-They put pressure on themselves (you work best when your back is against the wall.)

-They have routines, mighty discipline & healthy habits to maximize their output.

But most importantly, they are **consistent**.

'Dang & they still have time to handle other parts of their life?'

Yes. Because when this group rests, they **rest**.

They can rest knowing that they gave it their ALL during their work sessions. They rest by hanging with loved ones, watching a show, unwinding etc.

'But isn't taking rest sessions soft?'

Not at all. You need to be able to take rest sessions to keep your engine running smoothly. While group 1 burns out & questions why they feel miserable, group 2 plays for the long run & feels emotionally stable.

You need to be emotionally stable if you want to play for the long run. When the mind & emotions work in harmony, you build laser-like focus AND passion. That's why group 2 feels like they aren't even working. They are just having fun!

But don't mistake fun for weakness. Fun is what allows you to make MASSIVE progress. You need to enjoy what you do in order to leverage obsession.

Mighty focus + Rest sessions = Leveraging obsession to your favor.

No more looking like an extra from Walking Dead.

Now go! Begin to take your time more seriously. Make improvements in 2 months that it takes someone else 2 years to do.

Defy all odds.

Become obsessed.

How to Properly Execute Discipline

☆*Fit people were once fat.*

☆*Masters were once beginners.*

☆*Successful people were once failures.*

☆*Mature people were once immature.*

☆*Driven people were once lazy.*

You can make any change that you desire. The only thing standing in your way is discipline.

'I can make any change that I desire?'

Absolutely. You just need the discipline to make it happen.

'Is discipline really that important though?'

Yes. It is lifechanging. But understand one thing, discipline is not simply an act, it is a mindset.

'A mindset? I thought discipline just meant following a routine.'

And what do you think following that routine does? It alters your mindset.

An altered mindset = An altered reality

Sad truth is that a lot of people pussyfoot when it comes to discipline. They do it some days, neglect it on other days & soon abandon this life-changing principle. But that's because they are misguided.

To optimize disciple, you need:

A why

A how

A what

Desire = Why

Long term blueprint = How

Daily routine = What

The incorrect way to do it is to just jump into the 'what.' Poor strategy! Doing a bunch of random productive acts without the slightest clue as to why is a recipe for disaster & will lead to quitting. Here's how you correctly bring discipline into your world:

1. You need to start with your **WHY**. Why do you want to be disciplined?? Is it to get fit, become rich, become confident? Identifying you WHY engages your emotions. It awakens your DESIRE.

2. Visualize your **HOW**. This part will be hazy at first since you are just starting your journey. But visualizing & consistent action helps you cut thru the busy work & find out what really matters. You leverage your imagination to create a blueprint & then you carve out your path.

3. Do the **WHAT**. Once you have gone thru step 1 & 2, doing your daily routine will feel MUCH easier. Heck, it will even feel like fun! Why? Because you are now working with purpose rather than just throwing shit at the wall & seeing what sticks.

Direction > Speed

You see, my friend, you were mistaken all along. You have a LIMITING belief that says discipline is supposed to be boring. But in reality? Discipline is far from boring. It is *fulfilling*. If fulfillment doesn't excite you, then I don't know what to tell you.

Your wildest dreams can manifest into reality if you have the mental toughness to execute on your discipline. You need to be consistent, not just when you feel like it. That's what separates the winners from the losers.

Now go get what's yours. Don't let one single person stop you from getting it. But most importantly, don't let yourself stop you from getting it.

It all started with a thought.

The thought was repeated.

The thought was worked on.

As time passed, the thought became a behavior.

You worked more, day in & day out.

Soon, the behavior began producing results.

Is it magic?

No. It's consistency.

Consistency Will Awaken Your Inner Genius

They call it miracles. I just call it staying consistent for long enough. It's almost impossible not to get one W after a flurry of Ls.

The human brain is a powerhouse. Think about it for a second. How often did you get in your car, and after some time had elapsed, you were at your destination? You had just driven a car, but you did it so seamlessly that you didn't even notice it. Too many times to count I bet!

How is this even possible? It's because your brain has incorporated driving into its existence. You can automatically do the task on autopilot. But why stop at driving? Why not go past that & see what else you can do on autopilot?

That's where consistency comes in. The majority don't reach their goals because they have not been consistent. They do it one day, neglect it for a few days, come back to it, and they stay at a subpar level. Then they blame the task saying it's too hard! Laughable.

Just be consistent, do self-analysis & your brain will figure out the rest. Here is an exercise to make sure you remain consistent. And yes, this exercise is named after the legendary Jerry Seinfeld who practiced utilized this routine to write his standup routines.

Seinfeld Chain Strategy:

1. Identify the skill you want to learn.

2. Buy a calendar with all months on one page.

3. Buy a red sharpie.

4. Everyday practice the skill & mark a 'X' for the day.

5. Form the chain of X's & do not let it break.

Your skillset will solidify in no time.

The Difference Between Good Failure & Bad Failure

'How are failures good? It only wastes my time.'

It may waste your time now, sure. But then, the failures give you lessons. And those lessons save you time in the future.

I'm not a big fan of using the word 'failure' because it automatically forces a negative perception. But the word is necessary. It is necessary because it sparks action in humans. Throughout your level up journey, this word will begin to form a level of nuance. You'll learn that there are 2 kinds of failure: bad failing & good failing.

Bad failing is when you are failing the same exact way over & over again.

-You aren't learning from your mistakes.

Good failing is when you are failing in innovative ways.

-You are now gaining new data to eventually figure it all out.

189

You can't learn anything new if you refuse to fail. Failing is a byproduct of picking up something innovative. View failure as 'gathering data.' But once you gather the data, you need to analyze it. Otherwise, you are going from 'gathering data' back to failure.

As you are learning & executing in practicing these skills, you are going to be going thru a lot of trial & error.

But **patience**.

Each failure is a dot.

Stack up failures & extract the lessons.

With time, the dots will begin to connect.

The picture will blossom before your very eyes.

Till then, always show up & show out.

Resting like a Champion

In order to play for the long run, you need to work AND rest.

Overworking is no badge of honor. Heck, it is detrimental to your level up journey.

Have you ever had that moment where you are working nonstop for day, weeks, months? And as you are working & working, something very strange happens. You just shut down & go on a long lazy spree?

'That sounds very familiar.'

The reason for this phenomenon is because when you do not assign your body rest, it will assign it for you.

Understand that energy is limited, not limitless. You are not a machine who can work nonstop. And as an engineer who has worked with systems for many years, even machines are not always running. They are assigned downtime to preserve the engine. If machines need rest, then so do you.

My 2 rules of thumb regarding rest are very simple:

1. You earn your rest.

2. When you rest, you rest. Not rest, check your emails, rest, work etc.

By following this 2-step formula, you will be able to rest & be a more efficient worker. Honest truth? I will say that rest is JUST as important as working in the level up journey.

Make sure you do not neglect it & risk burnout.

How to Properly Teach

Teaching is powerful because you learn more by teaching others than you learn on your own.

When you have effectively learned a subject or skill, it is time to give back. It is time to find a student and teach them.

You should be doing the LEAST amount of work possible when teaching. Sit back, guide & let them make their own mistakes. That's how the student learns to think for themselves. Hand holding does **nothing**.

'So you're telling me less is more when it comes to teaching?'

Correct.

'Not sure if I'm following. I thought I should teach my mentees by telling them what to do.'

Completely wrong.

- When you are telling someone WHAT to think, it leads to dependency.

- When you are teaching someone HOW to think, it leads to independency.

193

It's difficult to tell the difference because in the school system, we are often told what to think. But you need to be very careful. Chances are you are a victim of this or causing someone to be a victim of this.

From here on out, when you are teaching someone something that you know very well, let your student do the work. Sit on your ass & let them make their own mistakes. Ask strategic questions to guide them when they're stuck. That's it.

And if someone is teaching you something, ensure they're not lecturing you the whole time. Take matter into your hands & ask to do more work for yourself.

When a human puts in work, their neural pathways begin to connect & solidify. That's how their brain digests concepts & begins using its own creativity to think for itself.

In summary, do less! We already know that you're a pro. No need to show off how smart you are. Give your student the chance to prove how smart they can become.

You'll feel extra proud when your mentee begins pulling off your lessons & adding their own twists to it. And now you have raised a student who can pass your wisdom off to the next student. Teaching 101.

Bonus: You leave smarter than you entered. That's how the game was meant to be played!

From the Student -> Creator -> Teacher

This section hopefully taught you the art of learning so you can produce results and teach others how to produce results. In order to level up and skyrocket your growth, you need to be a learning and producing machine.

At the end of the day, you will not be remembered for the opinions you had. You will be remembered for the results that you produced with your mind & heart. When you know how to learn & are learning something that you have a desire for, the self-education journey feels like a blast. You design your own life curriculum & find innovative ways to engineer your future.

We are living in the golden era of learning. So much information out there that can fuel you to greatness. Make the most out of it my friend. In order to conclude this chapter, I will leave you with a cheat code to help you think bigger picture.

CHEATCODE to leave a legacy:

1. Aim to become the best version of yourself.

2. Then aim to help people become the best version of themselves.

Note: The more lives you impact, the stronger your legend grows.

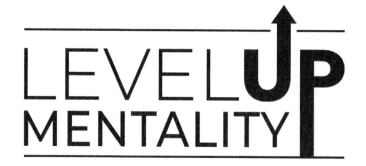

PART 7:

Dealing with
People

The Social Creature

At the very core, humans are social creatures. Back during our primal days, it was pretty much viewed as a death sentence when you were outcasted from your tribe. In today's world, I wouldn't say that the repercussions are that severe, however there are some.

With the rise in technology, social skills are scarce. Humans are now able to entertain themselves with their smart TV's, Netflix accounts, smartphones etc. Why bother leaving the house & meeting up with people in real life?

But this is a dangerous mindset to approach. No amount of technology & man-made entertainment will override the core of a human. Although we should not view it as a death sentence to work in isolation, we should still view it to be detrimental. For you to become your best self, it will not happen on its own.

Think about it for a second. I'm pretty sure you got to where you are today by having a few people helping you along the way. If you can close your eyes & take a walk down memory lane, you will most likely have at least 5 people that have played a big role in your present-day self. Very rarely will you see someone at the top of their field without any form of assistance.

Despite the good that comes with humans, there is also the bad. All humans are not going to have your best interest in mind. There will be many that want to do you harm. Haters & snakes, toxic people being a few of them.

Which is why it is so important to level up your social dynamics knowledge in order to navigate around the chaotic social world. The circle you surround yourself with can either level you up or level you down.

Let's make sure you don't fall into the latter category by engraining helping you learn the fundamentals of social dynamics. In this section, you will learn about your most precious currencies, the nice guy, how to form a tribe, deal with toxic people & much more.

Now let us enter the wonderful world of social dynamics.

Your Most PRECIOUS Currencies

Only give these currencies to high value people. Never spend these currencies on low value shit heads example: trolls, weasels, snakes, naysayers etc.

-Energy

-Time

-Attention

-Trust

-Love

-Loyalty

-Respect

'I thought money was the most important currency?'

Nope! There is no shortage of money in this world. Making the dollars your most important currency will have you leading an empty life. Time to flip your perspective.

· -**Energy**: When you strip yourself to the core, you are an emotional creature. Emotions are your internal worlds energy. Harnessing that energy is crucial for leveraging yourself to obtain whatever you want. You have a finite amount of energy every day, so spend it wisely.

-**Time:** A second that is lost will never be returned. You start valuing the hell out of this currency the more you mature. As the years start adding up, you realize time is precious. You must always have a scarcity mindset towards time. Once you do so, you will no longer be lazy.

-**Attention:** You can be here, but not present. Attention is completely mental. Giving someone your attention means you are clearing up mental bandwidth to make room for them. Only give your attention to people who help you grow. For the negative ones? Ignore their existence.

-**Trust**: People get bitten by so many snakes because they make their trust cheaper than Tootsie Rolls. Sad. The more you cheapen your trust, the more you invite toxic energy into your life. Make your trust expensive! Then make people earn it thru actions, not words.

-**Love:** You will give your love to many people in your life that do not value it. So what do they do? They do you dirty. But no matter what, always keep your head up. This emotion is powerful. Avoid the tendency to let past experiences jade your view of the invisible bond.

-**Loyalty**: The more you mature, the more loyal people will surprise you. You mature after you learned the dark truth about the real world. Most are disloyal. But avoid falling into the trap of being like them. Have UNBREAKABLE loyalty to the people who are loyal to you.

-**Respect:** The currency that is often misunderstood. People spend this precious currency on low value people. Nah. Never show respect to racists, haters, snakes etc. That doesn't mean to be disrespectful. Just distance yourself & give them 0 energy.

You see? These were the most important currencies all along. But society wants you to believe its money. That's a lie! When you are on your deathbed, you will not be thinking about your bank account.

You will be thinking about your: experiences, loved ones, the person you ended up becoming. That's what really matters. That's how you think big picture while everyone else is thinking small. Change your life forever. Adopt these currencies as the most important.

Spend these currencies on the right people, projects & events. And believe it or not, by doing this, the money will come.

Time to level up your reality.

The Difference between Nice & Kind

People come & go. The person across the mirror stays the same. You're going to be stuck with yourself forever. Start making yourself the priority.

Making yourself the priority is a lifechanging moment in the social dynamics world. Until you make this mental transition, you are going to always notice something very daunting. You are going to notice yourself being the 'nice guy.'

The nice guy is a people pleaser who changes their personality like they change their clothes. A few traits of the nice guy include:

-excessive giggling

–agreeing with every point

-switching your beliefs to agree with others

-shitty eye contact

-fidgeting nonstop

-saying sorry a lot

-ending every sentence with 'I think' etc.

You may be wondering why the nice guy behaves the way that he does. It is because he wants **approval**. He wants to be liked by others, so instead of making himself the priority, he makes others the priority.

'Do people end up liking him more?'

Nope. Exact opposite.

People become repulsed by the nice guy. Although the nice guy does & says all the right things, other humans simply do not feel comfortable around him. Their subconscious mind can tell something about all the niceness is fake.

This results in the other people taking advantage of the nice person & tossing them to the side.

Instead of being nice, be kind.

'I thought they were the same thing?'

Nope.

- Nice= Delivering a real message by accident or fake message + Positive delivery
- Kind = Delivering a real message + Positive delivery

Noticed that I said that a nice guy delivers a real message by accident. Because they don't care about delivering a real message or not. They are mainly focused on delivering a message for acceptance. If they do give a real message, it was typically by accident.

On the other hand, the kind guy is authentic. Their main intention is based around staying true to themselves & being real.

Often, we believe that being real means being an asshole. But that is not true. You can be real & polite at the same time.

And unlike the nice guy, the kind guy is respected by his peers! He sends off a calm, poised, authentic energy that has him attracting the right people into his life. While the nice guy doesn't like himself & others don't like him either, the kind guy is living a different life. The kind guy loves himself & others are now able to value him as well.

From here on out, make yourself the priority, and aim to be kind, not nice.

Why Authenticity is King

At the end of the day, you are a magnet. You attract what you put out there. Which is why it's dangerous to pretend to be someone that you're not. You begin magnetizing people who love the illusion of you, but do not really love the real you.

The social dynamics world is primarily based off energy. The energy that you put out there will be the energy that you attract. This concept is the main reason why you want to be authentic.

Being authentic is easier said than done. Why? Because in many cases, we often don't know who our authentic self really is. Humans are such nuanced creatures that it is difficult to pinpoint exact behaviors.

But the trick to finding and maximizing your authentic self is a 2-step process:

1. Analysis.
2. Talking to people like lifelong friends.

1. **Analysis** – In this step, I want you to find 3 people that you are very close with. Once you have identified them, I want you to analyze your mannerisms the next time you hang with them:

How are you behaving?

What are you talking about?

How do you feel?

Look out for underlying patterns. The patterns are the answers which shed light into your authentic self. Making yourself aware of the patterns is huge because it signals to your core self what is normal & abnormal for you. The next time you are acting like someone out of the ordinary, your awareness will signal to you that something is off. Once you have identified your authentic self, apply it.

2. **Talking to people like lifelong friends-** Apply your analysis from step 1 on this step. This is when you exercise your social muscle to be more comfortable in social settings. At first, you will feel a little uneasy showing the world your authentic self but understand that is part of the process.

You are now cutting thru the noise from the get-go. You are allowing the people who are not fond of your authentic self to excuse themselves from your life & keeping the ones who like you.

By being authentic, you attract the right people & are no longer putting on an act.

If you can exercise your mindset to fight thru the awkwardness, you will feel more comfortable in social interactions. You are exercising your authentic self to be your baseline behavior. Once you achieve that, you will become the magnet that attracts people who love you for the real you.

Finding a Tribe

'Butter knife sharpens iron.' Said no one ever. You can never reach greatness surrounded by bums.

'Iron sharpens iron.' Keep your circle packed with people who are hungry for success.

I am sure you have heard the saying, 'You are the average of your 5 best friends.'

And to no surprise, that saying is 100% true. The friends that you surround yourself with are having a bigger impact on your future than you can possibly imagine.

I remember a few years ago, I was hanging out with a bunch of losers, partying & entertaining a bunch of nonsense. To my 'surprise' I was shocked to see how it was affecting my life. Poor grades, more anxiety & playing catch up. But why?

It's because your friend circle spreads energy, the language of the subconscious mind. Remember, your subconscious mind see's life thru images & emotions. When you are surrounding yourself with losers, toxic people & victims, your subconscious mind is carefully watching and picking up the habits.

A few years later, I realized that my friend circle was not the best for me. So, I went monk mode & aimed to level up my life. During this level up journey, I picked up Toastmasters, wrapped up my engineering degree & worked out.

As I began to create value for myself, I went from chasing others, to attracting. A lot of people who were now entering my life were better suited to my values. And since building the new tribe, life has been much more efficient in the level up journey.

If you are looking to find your tribe, you need to be able to distinguish between a social asset & social liability.

Social Asset: A social asset is someone who empowers you. This person helps you on your level up journey to become your best self. Although you may have a different north star from your asset, they are working towards something trying to become better. A social asset needs to provide value. The value can come in terms of emotional support, helping you with a skill, someone to bounce ideas off etc.

Social Liability: A social liability is someone who drains you or brings out the worst in you. They provide you no value & tend to take you off your life path. They are typically seen in toxic relationships, someone who only gossips, a person without a life mission etc.

Once you can distinguish between a social asset & a social liability, you need to make it an effort to give 100% effort to social assets & 0% effort to social liabilities. Very simple principle that is often overlooked. In the level up journey, you can't be entertaining draining energy at all. Cut energy vampires off ruthlessly.

Now that you know the 2 main buckets of social groups, follow do the following:

Build your life.

Be social.

No need to overcomplicate it. Typically, both 1 & 2 will play off each other. As you are building your life in terms of chasing your north star, you will notice yourself crossing paths with a lot of like-minded people. Once you do, consciously focus on sparking up the conversation. Don't wait for them to come up to you & introduce themselves. Rather, take the active approach, break the ice & be social.

By doing this, you will notice that you are meeting a lot of new people. There is a catch to all of this. Meeting a lot of people is great & all, but you do not want to call them a friend so quick.

In order to level up, you need to be very choosy with who you consider a friend. Giving out the title of friend to everyone will have you devaluing the bond. You need to consider it an honor to be a part of your tribe. Make it an exclusive group by only selecting a handful of winners. Therefore, it is important to have a social filtration system. It goes something like:

Step 1: Network – At this stage, you are being social and meeting new people.

Step 2: Rapport building – At this stage, you are looking for commonalities or just trying to get to know more about the person.

Step 3: Acquaintance formed- At this stage, you have gotten to know the person well enough to exchange contact information & help each other out in the future. You 2 should be able to add value to each other's lives. Don't just go off making everyone an acquaintance!

Step 4: Friend formed- Only a select few should make it to this stage. This stage should consist of people that you can build a social & emotional connection with. But most importantly, they need to be loyal. Loyalty is a huge factor in building a tribe. One reason why I have always been a proponent of a small circle over a big one was due to the scarcity of loyalty in today's world. As you mature, you are not going to be more trusting, you are going to be less trusting. Be selfishly picky.

Once you have done the social filtration system, your phone will be filled with many more contacts!

Now pick and choose though the information to build your tribe! You don't have to limit yourself to only one tribe. I recommend having a few that help you level up in different facets of life.

One recommendation is having a tribe tier system:

Big tribe: Consists of many acquaintances & friends. This tribe is big & allows for you all to mastermind, share tips, promote each other's brands & life mission.

Middle sized tribe: Consists of some acquaintances & friends. This tribe is smaller & more personal. This allows for stronger social bonds & a place to bounce ideas off.

Exclusive tribe: Consists of only friends. This tribe is more personal & discusses exclusive topics not seen by the external world.

You have the personal freedom to form your tribe that best suits your life mission. Build a tribe full of winners & sharpen your mind in the process.

Social Bonds Formation 101

Break:

enter their world by introducing yourself.

Spark:

get to know each other.

Maintain:

exchange contact info for follow ups.

Strengthen:

follow up.

Reward Loyalty with Royalty

Look out for the people who looked out for you when you didn't have anything.

In the social dynamics world, your character is everything. A person without character is seen as a low social valued human by high social valued humans.

And if you are trying to level up, then you **need** people to take it to the next stage. Therefore, you want to guard your character by maximizing your loyalty.

Loyalty is the invisible bond that connects humans with one another. The sad thing is that loyalty is a scarce resource in today's world. We live in a social world full of haters, snakes & weasels.

When you see a loyal person, it becomes a breath of fresh air. But understand that you need to make your loyalty valuable. You make it valuable by doing the following:

1. **Reward loyalty with royalty.**

2. **Distance from the disloyal ones.**

I actually see people staying loyal to someone who has backstabbed them because they think it makes them a 'good person.'

Wrong.

It makes you a foolish person. You devalue your loyalty when you stay loyal to a disloyal person & you are rewarding bad behavior. As you are leveling up, you need to get a major concept thru your head:

You do not try to fix people who do not think there is anything to fix.

Just because you have the right intention for them does not mean you will rewire their subconscious mind. Give disloyal people nothing.

As for loyal people, give them the world. Loyal people will go thru hell & back to make sure you are leveling up as you should: 1 loyal friend beats 100 material possessions.

There will be plenty of temptations in the real world to break loyalty but value the invisible bond & never forget where you come from.

Your character is a lot more important than you can imagine, so guard it with life. Loyalty is a magnetic force in a tribe. As you grow as a person, it is much more fun to see others growing with you. Have your tribe member's back & stay alert to make sure they are doing the same for you.

The Difference between Character & Reputation

Character: you can always control.

Reputation: you can't always control.

Character is how you carry yourself & reputation is how other people perceive you.

'Which one should I focus on as I am leveling up?'

Focus on character.

'Why?'

Because unfortunately, the real world is not all butterfly & rainbows. There are 2 creatures that exist that will try to harm your reputation no matter how good of a person you are: haters & snakes.

Haters & snakes will gossip, talk shit & spread lies about you. And very often, other people will believe their words before confirming it with you. Is it fair? Not really. But you must accept reality for what it is, not what you wish it to be.

Which is why I recommend focusing on your character. Stay true to yourself & honor your life principles. From there, the right people will stay & the wrong people will leave.

You will always have the right reputation with the right people who are meant to be in your life if you carry yourself the right way. *Read that again.*

People who believe gossip about you without getting your side of the story were never loyal ones anyways. Let them kick rocks, you don't need them anyway!

Focus on your character & what you can control, then let the rest of the cards fall into place.

Haters = Losers

I've never met one hater that is doing better than the person they are hating on. That alone speaks volumes.

As you begin to level up, you will notice that you are attracting a lot more haters. It will typically come from strangers, family members, or even friends who you are outgrowing. But the people who hate on you are typically doing worse than you.

'If they are not doing better than the person they are hating on, why not work harder?'

Because that would require logic.

People who hate, react to their primal emotion of jealousy rather than respond.

Human process information with their emotional brain before their logical brain. Jealousy is a very primal response that every human feels. But what you DO with the emotion determines your value in society.

2 types of people:

Person A: Feels jealous. Assigns it a positive perception. Becomes inspired to do something about it.

Person B: Feel jealous. Assigns it a negative perception. Becomes a hating ass bitch in the process.

'What sparks jealousy?'

A hidden desire.

'Any examples?'

Say you see a kid making a lot of money online and you get jealous. That means a hidden desire of yours is to make more money as well. Sometimes, the desires are small, so it can be ignored. Sometimes, they are BIG.

As you rise in your field, you will spark MANY people's hidden desires. And the sad reality is that most humans assign a negative perception to their jealousy, becoming haters in the process.

'Should I be scared?'

Not at all.

You should feel honored.

'Why?'

Because losers do not spark jealousy in other humans, only winners spark jealousy. You're on the right path, keep moving forward.

Social dynamics Law:
In order to be loved by many, you need to be hated by many.

Which group are you going to place your focus on? The choice is yours.

But from here on out, change your attitude towards haters. Let the low social valued creatures hate, while you look down to chuckle at them from your throne. They aren't going to stop you. Heck, they will power you up even MORE.

Once it's all said and done, you will have produced results & will have forged a legacy. And for your haters? They will feel shame for how they behaved, just give it time.

CHEATCODE to thick skin:

You only get mad at haters when you assign them equal or higher social value.

Wrong.

Haters are born thru assigning themselves low social value.

Why hype them up?

LEARN THIS CONCEPT.

Your anger will turn into sympathy from here on out.

Magic.

Respecting your Time

Giving your time to people who disrespect you is silly. You only give them your time because your ego wants to clear its name & you have a scarcity mindset towards people. Fuck them & their opinions. Give your most scarce resource to people who you respect & give you respect.

Picture this for a second:

-Your life vision = North star

-Your journey = Your path

Every day, your goal is to move FORWARD on this path, so you edge closer to your north star. Moving forward comes in many shapes & sizes. Here are a few:

-educating yourself

-executing your ideas

-connecting with other like minds

Level Up Mentality

-taking care of your health so you play for the long run

With all these tasks that you have on your plate, what good does giving your time to a hater do for you? When you give your time to a hater, you stop moving forward on your path & actually start walking backwards!

'So why do so many people give haters their time?'

Plenty of reasons, some being:

-untamed ego

-weak north star

-poor emotional control

-scarcity mindset towards people.

-**Untamed ego**: When your ego is untamed, you take shit personally. But remember, how others view you is how they view themselves. It's rarely about you.

-**Weak north star:** When your life purpose is weak, you tend to get distracted a lot. Take some time to re-evaluate your north star. Right now, you're lacking desire. Find out why.

-**Poor emotional control:** You react to disruptive emotions like a chump. Train your mind to be stronger than your emotions.

-**Scarcity mindset towards people:** When you have this mindset towards people, haters sound very loud. But understand that there are BILLIONS of people on this planet. Adopt abundance mentality towards people, then haters will sound like whispers.

Whichever category you fall in, understand that time is one of your most precious resources. If you're going to have a scarcity mindset towards anything, it *needs* to be your time.

Stop giving your time to people who disrespect you! Mute them on social media & mute them in real life. Exercise your self-control skills. Not every situation needs words. Ignoring is a response in itself, and a VERY powerful one at that.

Why Ignoring Beats Attacking Back

Ditch the 'attack back' mentality.

-shows little self-control & will have you feeling drained.

Adopt the 'ignore' mentality.

-shows more self-control & will not have you feeling drained.

'I thought attacking them back showed that I was a boss?'

No boss would condone of your behavior.

'Why? Isn't ignoring the cowardly thing to do?'

Not at all, it shows power. Let me explain it with some social dynamic's concepts.

People who attack others do it because they lack self-esteem. You will rarely see someone who is making major moves in their life take the time to pick on others. They simply do not have the time. But low social valued creatures? They have all the time in the world.

225

Low self-esteem + A lot of free time = Poison

These people can be poisonous in many ways. But often, their method of choice is to name call & stir up shit with people who they view to be a higher social value. So, they attack. Now you have 2 options:

Option 1. Attack Back

Many high social value people fall for this trap. They believe it is the 'powerful' thing to do. 'Let me put this hater in place!' they say. But this option is a very poor choice.

'Why is it poor?'

Because it gives the low social valued person what they want.

'And what is that?'

Attention.

You see, any form of attention from a high social valued person is seen as a reward to a low social valued person. Good or bad. If you attack them back, they will give themselves a pat on the back for getting a reaction out of you.

These losers have 0 other things going on in their lives, so they become the Energizer bunny when they get people to snap at them. And guess what? You just took an L. You have now strayed off your life mission to entertain this clown. And guess what?

'What?'

They'll do it again. And you will attract other haters coming at you hoping you give them attention as well. Very annoying process to be stuck in and highly distracting. You end up feeling drained. The drained energy begins to negatively perform your output.

Option 2. Ignore

Ignoring requires a lot of self-control. Why? Because you are forced to tame your ego. The ego naturally wants to attack back when it feels disrespected. Which is why taming it is no easy task, but well worth it. It is worth it because:

1. You starved the low social valued creature of attention, which will drive them insane. Very funny to witness, so you get a good chuckle out of it.

2. But more importantly, you preserve your energy. This is all energy that you can channel to knock your goals out the park.

Let me ask you something. When you go shopping for clothes, do you:

1. Buy an item you like.

2. Buy an item you like AND another item you don't like.

'Obviously option 1.'

Why?

'Because why spend my money on something I don't like? Option 2 is stupid.'

Exactly!

Now ask yourself, why spend your TIME + ENERGY on someone you don't like? The answer is, you don't! Let them think whatever they want to think. Let them throw a hissy fit begging for your attention. Those clowns are not your concern whatsoever. Your only concern is your mission.

The next time you want to clap back, ask yourself: Am I gaining anything from giving my time & energy to this individual? If not, then keep it moving! You'll feel **much** better in the process.

Make them irrelevant > Hold a grudge

Holding a grudge is the easy thing to do.

But holding a grudge is not the right thing to do.

A grudge puts poison in your body & rewires your subconscious mind.

You consume the poison & destroy your reality while your attacker sleeps like a baby.

Making the attacker irrelevant is a superpower that a few have mastered.

When you make an attacker irrelevant, it crushes their soul.

They did their best to get a reaction out of you, but nothing?

Being deemed irrelevant puts poison in their body & consumes them.

They try to attack more hoping to get any crumbs of attention.

But you maintain your power & elevate yourself.

Now it is you who sleeps like a baby while their head is spinning in circles.

That's how the game was meant to be played.

Hold the grudge = you lose & they win.

Make them irrelevant = you win & they lose.

Which option are you going to choose after reading this?

Your choice will say a lot about how much of a control you have over your ego.

Choose wisely.

How to Deal with Snakes

You may be wondering what is the difference between a hater & a snake?

- A hater is loud with their disdain towards you.
- A snake is quiet with their disdain towards you.

In many ways, this makes you sort of respect a hater more. At least the hater is honest & now you know that you aren't going to give them any of your time. But with a snake, they lie & pretend to be your friend.

I'll be honest with you... You are going to have to deal with a lot of snakes as you go on your level up journey. Is it fair? Not at all. But then again, the social dynamics world is not fair.

A snake comes in 2 forms:

1. Snake for a while.
2. Became a snake thru jealousy.

Part 1 deals with the kind of people who have always been a snake. They haven't had honor in most of their relationships. These people are the kings of backstabbing.

Part 2 deals with people who switch up on you. This one really hurts your soul. They probably have seen you thru a lot of good & bad moments in your life.

But as you kept leveling up, their jealousy for you grew. They didn't want to say anything because they viewed you as a friend for so long. But their jealousy became louder & louder before it began to consume them. Many would use their jealousy to identify what's making them jealous and chase that goal. But not the snake.

They decide to backstab you instead.

Getting bitten by a snake is never easy, I get it. I have had to deal with my fair share of snakes since beginning my journey.

But once someone shows you their true colors, you do **not** try to repaint them.

One way to get it wrong is by giving too many second chances. You need to be selective with your second chances, otherwise, you are going to git bitten left and right.

'Is there a framework to follow for how to give second chances?'

Yep. By being able to distinguish between a mistake & malice.

- Mistake is when someone did not have bad intent towards you.
- Malice is when someone did have bad intent towards you.

With mistakes, it is okay to give a second chance, but don't overdo it. If you are dealing with someone who makes the same repeated 'mistakes,' then it is no longer a mistake, it is a behavior. And associating with bad behavior is not something you want to be surrounded by in your level up journey.

Level Up Mentality

With malice, in my opinion, it is not okay to give second chances. Especially giving chances overnight! I see people who forgive a backstabber the next day, after they hear some sweet words.

But understand that humans do not change overnight. More often than not, the snake is coming back to you with their best behavior hoping for forgiveness. Once you forgive, they will remain in their best behavior for a certain period, until they go back to their old ways.

Now I do understand that humans are nuanced creatures. I do think people are capable of change. If someone comes back into your life after a long period of time & you genuinely want to give them another chance, then make your decision based off your own life. However, follow one tip: **focus on actions over their words**.

Don't let the good ole' days mentality creep up on you.

Snake bites will toughen your skin. Betrayal is never fun, but it will teach you more life lessons than a book ever will.

Extract the lessons from the experiences & apply it onto the future. You will learn how to move more fluidly in the social world.

Stop Taking Things Personally

'How do I stop taking things so personally?'

By understanding that people do not do stuff because of you. They do stuff because of themselves.

How they feel about you is dictated by how they feel about themselves. Making this realization helps you out tremendously in life.

You are now going to be able to deal with 2 of life's biggest challenges.

1. Criticism

2. Rejection

These are 2 parts of life that you need to be able to deal with. If you are leveling up, you are going to see it more than ever.

'What if I decide to remain a loser?'

Don't matter homie. You will be criticized & rejected for being a loser.

'Are you saying that I'm not the only person in the world who gets criticized & rejected?'

Correct. Every SINGLE human on the planet goes thru it as well. But there's a catch.

'And what's that?'

Rejection & Criticism forms 2 Groups:

1. **Losers**: energy gets drained, self-esteem suffers & they typically quit.

2. **Winners**: energy remains unaffected, self-esteem remains unaffected & they continue.

I spent many years as a loser. And many others start off as a loser as well. However, after a long time, the loser is met with a fork in the road.

-Remain a loser OR take the path of a winner.

This all ties back to the initial concept of not taking things personally. Once you learn the art of not taking things personally, taking the path of a winner becomes a no brainer. Why remain a loser when most of the fears are made up in your head?

The mental transition is not easy by any means. But it is worth it. Rejection & criticism will NEVER go away. Train your internal world to overpower any rocks that the external world throws at you.

The more goals that you cross off your list, the less opinions or comments from the external world will affect you. Just keep moving forward & keep your eyes on the prize at all times. You are only responsible for your actions, not other people's perceptions.

From here on out, start viewing rejection & criticism as a workout for your internal world.

Back to the drawing board.

Turn Sensitivity into a Compass

'Why did that person offend me?'

Wrong question! Instead, ask yourself 'why did I allow it to bother me?'

You'll get more insight into your internal world by asking the second question.

'Why do I get more insight with the second question?'

Because now you are bringing the focus back onto yourself. There is a reason that you're getting offended & it's time to find out why. Let me ask you something...

If I were to call you an alien as an insult, would you get offended?

'No.'

Why?

'Because I know it's not true.'

So why do you get offended when someone calls you a loser?

237

'Uh...'

Exactly.

You get offended because you have some self-doubts about yourself at times. Maybe not in front of other people, but during your alone time. Which is why being called a loser gets under your skin.

Asking the second question forces you to come to terms with your insecurities. Which is why you should view getting offended as signs for introspection rather than an opportunity to lash out.

Lashing out is easy, which is why most people do it. Coming to terms with certain insecurities is hard as fuck, which is why most people run away from it. But guess what?

You need to become immune to the words of others. If you know it's not true, let them think whatever they want to think. And if you lowkey know there is some truth to their harsh words, then show the courage to face that truth. But throwing a hissy fit gets you nowhere.

Remember the famous mantra grasshopper:

'The thicker the skin, the less the stress.'

The next time you're offended, be less angry & more curious! Guarantee this little mental flip will alter your reality.

You my friend, have turned a negative situation into a great opportunity for growth.

Play Chess While They Play Tic Tac Toe

Learn the art of noticing & not being vocal about it. This is how people who see the game 10 steps ahead, move. They understand that everything doesn't require a response. Strategic silence is deadly. This group notices, makes necessary adjustments & keeps it moving.

'Do you have an example of when strategic silences are used?'

In spotting human intentions.

Every human out there has an intention. Their intentions for themselves are crystal clear. They want the best for themselves. But with you? That's where their intentions get hazy.

Their intentions fall into one of the 3 categories:

-They are indifferent towards you.

-They want the best for you.

-They want the worst for you.

239

'Why is it important to use strategic silences when spotting human intentions?'

Because once they are aware that you are observing them, they will be on their best behavior. Even if that behavior is fake.

Which is why the silence allows you to notice their baseline actions towards you. Those baseline actions give insights into the persons internal world.

'Wait! Do people know when I'm lying to them?'

A lot of times, socially intelligent people will be able to tell. They have a great connection with their gut & are fluent in body language. But they choose not to say anything.

They want to see how creative you get with your lie. They want to see why you are lying in the first place. They are gathering more data about your intentions. So they remain silent & let you speak on....

Once they have their data, they know how to plan out their next moves.

'Why don't they confront me?'

Why should they? So you can lie some more? Ha! They don't have that kind of time for a weasel.

But this is just one of many usages of a 'strategic silence.' *It's when a human weighs the pros & cons of a situation, then decides whether words are necessary. If not, silence will be leveraged.*

Level Up Mentality

Give this move a try as you are filtering your social circle. See the game 10 steps ahead.

Play chess while they play tic tac toe.

Being Socially Dynamic

Hopefully in this chapter, you have gotten a clearer understanding on how to use social bonds to help you in your level up journey. Humans can serve as a vehicle for growth or an anchor as you try to become your grandest self. Which is why it is crucial that you understand human nature and make your moves wisely.

You will learn a lot more of your personal social dynamics principles as you continue in your journey. By becoming like water in the real world, you are able to see which humans are social assets & which ones are social liabilities. By being able to tell the difference between the two, you will be able to skyrocket your happiness, confidence & growth along the way.

Life is a lot better when you have good people around you to build memories with. Aim to always be social, then use your judgment to make sure you are attracting winners & repelling the losers.

Within time, you will stop being rigid & will be able to adapt like a social superstar. You will go from an ice cube to water. Till then, keep putting yourself out there & be social.

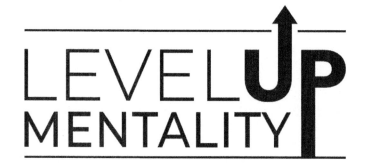

PART 8:
Creating
a Legacy

If you write it down,
you will soon become it.

Just watch.

Journal who you want to become
every day of your life.

Force yourself to level up daily.

Watch yourself blossom into a legend.

What is a Legacy?

Understand that greatness comes with a price.

'Like?'

Like:

Burned money

Sleepless nights

Failed relationships

Missed social events

Showing up even when you don't feel like it

Endless self-doubt

Endless haters

But you will still rise. Ready?

'Absolutely. Let's get it.'

Level Up Mentality

When you fight for a legacy, you fight for something bigger than yourself. Anyone can reach goals. The question is, what kinds of goals are you reaching?

That is why the level up mentality forces you to think in terms of legend or bust status. Aiming to create a legacy forces you to venture past your comfort zone & aim to unlock a different side of you. The side that holds greatness.

Becoming a legend is often misunderstood. It is seen as an unattainable goal because of how intimidating the word sounds. But if you break it down, it is **absolutely** possible.

A legend is an icon in a particular field.

Being an icon in a particular field is possible when you are able to have a north star in your life.

I remember a few months ago, I was hanging out with a few of my friends who had recently started a consulting business. And in the discussion, the name Sam Ovens popped up.

As soon as it did, a bunch of the people in the group were talking about how he is a legend. How his concepts have changed up their entire life & mindset. They couldn't stop talking about how this Sam Ovens fellow. They said that Sam will forever be regarded as a legend in their eyes.

That conversation ended up sparking my curiosity. I decided to do some research on Sam Ovens. Who was he & why did he incite such a strong reaction from my friends?

I Googled him & eventually stumbled onto his YouTube channel. The dude was only 29 years old!! How could he possibly be considered a legend??

But I dug deep into his content & I noticed an underlying pattern. This man was gifted. He wasted no time talking about fluff in his videos. He gave actionable mindset, online business & consulting tips. After watching 3 of his videos, I could confidently say that he changed my mindset towards money.

The next day, I went up to my cousin who had just starting an ecommerce business and asked him if he knew who Sam Ovens was. My cousin had no clue who Sam was or what he did.

And at that point, everything clicked! Sam Ovens was a legend to a particular group, not the entire world. Why? Because he had enhanced the lives of a certain group of people on this planet with his skillset.

He created a north star for his life, went on a journey to chase it, became a grander version of himself, then decided to give back. That is how a legend is born.

You don't need to appeal to the entire world. Because if you try appealing to everybody, then you will appeal to nobody. Your goal is to chase your north star, become the best version of yourself & then give back to the people who are chasing similar things as you are.

When you fight for a legacy, your efforts are not only impacting you, but your future generations, parents, friends & much more.

Level Up Mentality

That is what leveling up is all about. Without chasing a legacy, you will reach a ceiling & begin to stagnate.

But when you do chase a legacy?

You will become immortal.

The Light Bulb, Phone, TV & Airplane

You ever thought about a lot of the inventions that are present in today's world? The lightbulb, phone, TV, airplane being a few that come to mind.

What exactly made people create these devices? I'm sure they must have been viewed as crazy by their peers when they were going out of their way to build these tools. Let's use the airplane as an example.

How do you think that conversation went? 'Hey guys, my brother & I are going to create a vehicle that flies in the sky. Wish us luck!'

I'm pretty sure everyone looked at the Wright Brothers like they had 4 heads & then some. So what made them continue?

Why did they opt to build this device when it was viewed to be impossible?

*For one main reason: **Imagination**.*

They saw something that no one else could. Each of the inventors of the devices that I mentioned above saw something that was past the scope of society. While society was seeing the dots, these inventors were seeing the picture.

Level Up Mentality

Although society must have viewed them to be crazy whack jobs, the inventors must have viewed themselves as something more.

Years have gone by since their inventions have been designed. And who are we talking about now, the detractors or the creators?

We are talking about the creators because they leveraged their imagination. They were the ones who showed guts & turned the impossible to possible.

Incredible.

Could it be that imagination is one of the missing puzzle pieces to greatness? From these inventors & inventions, that certainly seems to be the case. But let's delve deeper into the brain to analyze the importance of imagination. Continue on...

The Left Brain & Right Brain to Create a Legacy

You have a logical side & a creative side. Your creative side is ingrained within you & your logical side is taught.

Let's take a walk down memory lane. When you were a kid, what kind of person were you, imaginative or logical?

'Imaginative.'

Did anyone teach you how to imagine?

'Nope, it just happened on autopilot.'

Exactly. You didn't see action figures. You saw actual characters due to your imagination breathing life into the inanimate. When did the logical side start kicking in?

'As I got older, went to school & started stacking up life experiences.'

Exactly. It was learned over time.

The two sides of a human are powerful. But unfortunately, a lot of humans only cap out on one side. In the school system and in society, we are not taught to harness our inner creativity. Rather, we are pounded with nonstop logic.

We are told to learn about subjects that we do not care about just so we can pass a test to see how logically we can apply it. And we go on years & years like this in the school system. What begins to happen? We begin to think like robots & our imaginative side takes a back burner.

But you can never kill what is ingrained. Your imagination is a part of you just like your emotions are. Which is why unused imagination turns into a different kind of monster.

When you simply think in terms of logic, your unused imagination begins to pair with the 'negativity bias' to build anxiety.

The negativity bias is your brain's natural proclivity to place more importance on the negatives over the positives.

You ever wondered why you have so much negative thoughts preplanning your failures? Those failures have never happened, so how are you seeing it in so much detail?

That is because your imagination is at work. Your imagination allows you to make eye contact with the impossible, *good or bad*.

- When you neglect to use your imagination, you will get anxiety.
- When you leverage your imagination, you will build a legacy.

How to make both brains work together

I am not trying to vilify logic by any means. Logic is going to come in handy in your journey. However, you can't be the person who ONLY uses logic. That will cause you to limit your thinking.

What you need to do is lead with creativity & verify with logic. Think of the inventors of our past generation. Everything that we have at our disposal was born from an idea. And this idea was then executed on, fine-tuned & created.

- Use your right brain (imaginative side) to think of innovative ideas & 10x the goals that you are chasing.
- Use your left brain (logical side) to design structured plans to bring those ideas to life.

That doesn't mean that you can't do something that someone else is doing. But do it bigger & better! You're not going to be a pro from the get-go, but make sure that you're keeping your brain thinking big at all times.

Example-

Wrong: I want to be the best writer in my city.

Right: I want to be the best writer in the universe.

In the wrong example, you are thinking too logically. In the right example, you are thinking imaginatively. And once you engage your imagination, you engage your emotions in the process. The subconscious mind is not a logical being, it is an emotional one. That is the mind that dictates 95% of your reality. Which is why you need the subconscious mind by your side when you're chasing a legacy. Think BIG.

Once you have thought big & identified your big goals, break them down! By breaking those goals down, you are now using your conscious mind to engage your logic. The logic will help you define deadlines, plans & routines to help you achieve your high-level goal.

With this method, you are utilizing your right brain & left brain in harmony. While all your other peers are thinking as logically as possible, you are thinking on a much bigger realm.

That is how you make both brains work together to carve out your own unique path towards a legacy.

Chronicling Your Level Up Journey

The Level up journey is the modern-day hero's journey that you read in books. You know, those books that go something like:

1. Everything is going well for the character.

2. Something goes wrong.

3. The character tries to make it right.

4. Character either succeeds or fails.

5. Leaves with lessons.

Obviously, your story is going to be much more complex & nuanced than that, but this is just a rough idea. When you have the potential to create your own life story, you begin to have a completely different viewpoint of life. You begin to view yourself as a hero that has much more control. You view your conflicts as challenges that will be conquered. You view your tribe members as unique characters that help you in this journey. You view your location as settings that you can choose at will.

Listen up my friend, this is a journey that **needs** to be chronicled. You may view the chronicling portion as a waste of time but hear me out.

Chronicling your journey does a few things:

1. You can see how far you have come.
2. You hold yourself accountable to keep moving forward.
3. You can release your journey to inspire people around the world.

Your life is one big story if you can view it that way. Chronicling your rise to the top is how you can view one of the *greatest* stories ever created.

Ways to Chronicle Your Journey

Luckily in today's world, there are an abundance of methods to chronicle your level up journey.

You can do it a few ways:

1. Private
2. Public
3. Both

1. **Private** is when you have you keep your journey to yourself. Picture journaling on your downtime.
2. **Public** is when you chronicle your journey to the world, so they can stay updated with your progress & you can form a tribe along the way.
3. **Both** is when you implement 1 & 2. There are certain things that you wish to keep private, so you jot it down on your own time. But there are certain things that you don't mind sharing, so you let the world take a peak as well.

Methods to Chronicle

1. **Journal**- You write about your past, present & future.
   a. Twitter.
   b. Blog.
   c. Word document.
   d. Physical journal.

2. **Audio Journal** – You talk about your past, present & future.
   a. Audacity + USB Microphone. This method allows you to create a podcast.
   b. Voice recorder in your phone.
3. **Video Journal** – You record about your past, present & future.
   a. YouTube channel.
   b. Video diaries on your laptop.

Whatever method you choose, aim to get it done. Recording the journey as it is playing out is a story that you will never get in a movie. Why? Because you are living it out for yourself! Having your story written will make it much more fulfilling when you are getting closer to your north star.

The beauty of it all? You can one day pass it onto your future generation so they can see how you blossomed into a legend.

Beautiful.

Final Thoughts About The Level Up Journey

When you buy a book, what do you do?

'Read it from the beginning.'

Why not the end?

'Because I need to go thru the journey to get to the end.'

Exactly. Same with life. The end will one day come. But first, you must go thru the journey.

The level up mentality will help a lot of people make sense of their lives. This is a structured mental framework that will optimize your happiness & challenge you to venture past your comfort zone.

As you are leveling up, make sure you are taking it day by day & enjoying the process. We are in such a rush to get everything done & over with, that we rarely enjoy the present day. But consciously focus on making sure that you are taking the time to enjoy the level up journey.

Level Up Mentality

You are taking a path in life that many people are too scared to take or are unaware of! Consider this as a rite of passage to become your grandest self.

In your journey, you will feel a lot of dark emotions, be dealt a lot of failures & deal with a lot of criticism. However, you will also learn a lot about yourself, shatter one goal at a time & meet several of cool people along the way. As the time flies by, you are going to see what a magical moment it is when you just compete against yourself & ignore competing against the world.

At that moment, you will realize that you were your only competition, harshest critic & best friend all along. It is time that you begin chasing your north star & leveling up to become your grandest self. This is a decision that will forever spark off Chapter 1 in the greatest story ever.

Good luck my friend.

Enjoy your level up journey.

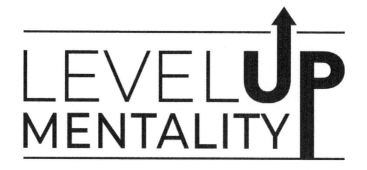

Bonus Part 1:

Life Laws
& Lessons

My Personal Life Lessons

In this bonus section, I have written down a lot of the lessons that I have learned along my journey. These are lessons that were learned the hard way. Take a look & see which ones you can apply to your story as well. Even if we are chasing a different north star, you will be shocked by how many things you are able to relate with.

Use the lessons that are applicable to your life & use it clarify your mindset.

The Trinity

-*Make your character so expensive that it cannot be bought.*

-*Make your time so scarce that it is never wasted.*

-*Make your emotional currency the money that you never spend on low value people.*

1. **Expensive character** Throughout your life, you will be presented with many temptations. Many times, you will give in. It happens, we are human. But use it as a lesson to not repeat the same mistake in the future. Guard your character with your life. Do not let yourself down.

2. **Scarce Time** Always have scarcity mentality with time. 'Each second you lose is each second you never gain back.' Once you truly understand this concept, you will begin to make the most out of your life. Use your time wisely, or regret your error in judgment later in life

3. **Emotional Currency** As you get older, you will start thinking in terms of energy. Reward people who match your energy with your emotional currency. If they are a different wavelength, give them nothing. Do not let a hater, snake, racist get a reaction out of you.

Life Laws Part 1.

If it angers you, it controls you.

If it hurts you, it toughens you.

If it scares you, it teaches you.

If it empowers you, it fuels you.

If it drains you, it poisons you.

☆ If it angers you, it controls you.

You are in charge of your emotions. You have the key. But when you give the key to someone else, then you have lost power. You have lost control. Be better. Hold on the key with life.

☆ If it hurts you, it toughens you.

A smooth sea never made a skilled sailor. You are going to get backstabbed, lied to, manipulated, dumped etc. But don't let the temporary hurt stop you. Introspection leads to the pain healing. Healed pain = Mental toughness

☆ If it scares you, it teaches you.

Fear is a compass. If you are scared of something, then it's teaching you more about yourself. It means you should do it. No need to overcome the fear overnight. Rather, do it over time.

☆ If it empowers you, it fuels you.

Do something that makes you feel alive. Be around people that make you feel alive. Your body holds a lot of your answers. Tune into it!! Feel the energy. Find what empowers you.

☆ If it drains you, it poisons you.

Stop arguing so much. Stop giving snakes second chances. And mute haters. You get to channel your focus on what you desire. Don't waste it on poison now. Be more calculated with your moves.

Life laws allow you to stay on track. It allows you to add clarity to ambiguity. Clarity allows you to choose your direction. Forward or backward?

The choice is yours.

The Power of Traveling

Traveling is primal. That's why you feel so refreshed after you visited somewhere you have never been. You think our primal ancestors were cooped up in their houses all day? Nah. They explored. Do the same. Travel the world one spot at a time.

It's very easy to get caught up in the level up journey that you begin to forget other parts of your life. One major facet being, traveling.

The power of travel goes beyond the traditional platitudes you hear regarding how it's an excellent vehicle to unwind. But I would go as far as to say that it is a primal act. It is in our core to want to travel & be where we have never gone.

Most people that are starting a business or a side hustle are not simply doing it for the money. They are doing it for the freedom. And along with the freedom comes the desire to explore.

Ask yourself where was the last place you visited? If you can't recall, then it's possible that you are getting too caught up in the work life.

I highly recommend that if you are someone going through a dark emotional time or if you are someone who has been feeling out of it lately, then get out there & travel somewhere new! And when you do travel, don't stay cooped up in the hotel room all day. But rather make it an effort to go out, try some new cuisines & sight see.

Make it an effort to visit at least one new place every year.

Tough, but doable.

Life Laws Part 2.

✫ When you are angry, distance.

Respond, don't react. Often, you will say some stuff in a heated moment that you wish you can take back. Save yourself the hassle. Distance, cool off & take it from there.

✫ When you are bored, learn.

You are living in the most advanced age of human civilization. There is no time to be bored. If you have nothing to do, go on & open a book. Follow your curiosities.

✫ When you are anxious, do.

Anxiety = Overthinking & under doing. If you feel anxious, get up & get active. Watch the nervous energy turn into productive fuel real quick.

✫ When you are sad, introspect.

Sadness is a powerful human emotion that sparks growth. Use your moments of sadness as an opportunity to look within. Introspect. You'll learn more about yourself in darkness than light. Know this.

✩ When you fail, analyze.

Unless you want to keep making the same mistakes over & over, then you need to analyze. Learn from what you did wrong so you can start doing right.

✩ When you win, win more.

Winning should not allow you to get content. Winning should fuel your ambition to win more. Be grateful for the accomplishments that you have stacked up. But keep your eyes forward. You still got more glory to chase.

2 Ways to Deal
with Rock Bottom

When life kicks your ass, there are 2 things that will not judge you:

-the weights

-your pencil & paper

Going to the gym & writing will help you heal your mind, emotions & spirit.

'Are you telling me that if I'm going thru rock-bottom right now, that these 2 acts will help me?'

Yes.

'Any idea why these acts are so effective?'

Yep, let me explain so you can do the acts with full confidence & consistency

When you are in turmoil, you will spend a lot of time in your head. But spending too much time in your head will self-destruct you, especially when you are going thru rock bottom.

Which is why you need to do 2 things:

1. An act that brings you to the present.

2. An act that allows you to make sense of your inner turmoil.

1. The weights bring you to the present. Heavy weights that challenge your strength will make you go from:

-mindless -> mindful mode

Plus, after your session, your brain will release endorphins, making you feel better.

2. The pencil & paper allows you to make sense of the internal turmoil. Don't care if you're a good writer or not. Just write. No one is watching. The more you write, the more you can bring clarity to the roller coaster emotions. Highly therapeutic when you get into the flow.

These 2 acts will speed up your recovery. But more importantly, it will help you become reborn.

'Reborn?? What are you talking about?'

You, my friend, are USING your pain. In the level up world, we use pain to produce. We do NOT let pain force us to go on a downward spiral.

There's a lot of things in this life that will lie to you. But the weights + paper & pencil? They will always tell the truth. These 2 exercises will lead to one final side effect. A side effect that will change your life forever. You will become best friends with yourself. And becoming best friends with yourself = true confidence.

Now begin.

Only you will be able to pull yourself out of rock bottom. Once you pull yourself out of the depths of hell, you will realize how powerful you were all along.

Weights + Pencil & Paper combo = Lifechanging

Do not miss your opportunity to use your pain as fuel.

Good luck.

Life Laws Part 3.

Immature = emotions overpowers mind.

Mature = mind overpowers emotions.

Socially unintelligent = talks more than listens.

Socially intelligent = listens more than talks.

Cocky = cares to be liked.

Confident = doesn't care to be liked.

Abundance mentality towards time will have you being lazy.

Scarcity mentality towards people will have you being needy.

Scarcity mentality towards time will have you being driven.

Abundance mentality towards people will have you being bold.

Learn to apologize without justifying.

Learn to turn down events without apologizing.

Learn to disagree without making an enemy.

Learn to critique without hating.

Learn empathize without coddling.

The 27 Lessons

In light of my 27th birthday, I would like to share 27 lessons that I have learned on my journey. A lot of these lessons were learned the hard way. But better late than never. Let's begin.

1. Chase experiences over material possessions.

2. Finding a life purpose will turn your life from scary & boring -> fun & challenging.

3. Have more compassion towards others. Many people are fighting a silent battle that you may have no clue about.

4. Learn the hard skills, then level up to soft skills when ready.

5. The person who broke your heart did you a massive favor. A few of the most valuable life lessons will be found behind a heartbreak.

6. Loyalty is scarce in today's superficial world. Snakes are abundant.

7. Understand that as you are growing older, so are your parents. Give them more attention & love.

8. A small well vetted circle who supports you is better than a big circle that brings in drama.

9. Meditation & journaling connects you to your internal universe.

10. Take care of your body by working out, eating well & doing yoga.

11. Do not get so caught up in work that you neglect your loved ones.

12. Anyone is prone to switching up on you. Therefore, you must learn to become your best friend. Always have your back.

13. You need to feel very lost in life before stuff eventually begins to click.

14. When learning a new skill, practice it slowly. You need to do it mindfully before you can do it mindlessly.

15. Call people more often to just catch up.

16. Once you have reached the bar you set for yourself, raise it even higher, then reach it again. Do this forever.

17. Mastering your emotions is the true sign of intelligence. Not some man made test.

18. Watch more interviews of legendary figures. Hear their blueprint.

19. Forgive & remember. Forgive so you can move on. Remember so you don't fall for the same trap again.

20. Debating is a waste of time if you are to chasing a legacy.

21. Do not attack back at your haters, instead MASTER the art of ignoring.

22. It often takes a loss of a life to truly appreciate the value of a life. But do not let this be the case. Show love to the loved ones.

23. Be more selfish & invest in yourself, so one day you can be selfless & give back.

24. Embrace your pain & use it to fuel the ambition.

25. Always make time to travel & try new cuisines.

26. Miracles are possible for everyone. You just need to be consistent long enough.

27. It is never too late to turn your life around for the best. You are a few good habits away from being reborn.

Alphabet of Life

My Alphabet of Success:	Alphabet of Failure:
Ambition	Average
Boldness	Backstabber
Charisma	Coward
Dependable	Disrespectful
Empathetic	Egotistical
Failures	Fearful
Grit	Grumpy
Honor	Hypocrite
Intellect	Impatient
Journey	Jealous
Kindness	Killjoy
Losses	Lazy
Mission	Messy
Nurturing	Negligent
Opportunities	Obnoxious
Patience	Procrastinator
Quality	Quitter
Resilient	Racist
Solitude	Stubborn
Teamwork	Trashy
Unique	Unhappy
Victory	Victim mentality
Wholesome	Whining
X-factor	Xenophobe
Yearn	Yeller
Zen	Zombie minded

6 Months = Magic Number

If you're going thru a tough time right now, I'm telling you.... Just 6 months.

That's all it takes to MASSIVELY turn your life around forever.

I'm speaking from experience.

Life doesn't have to be this way for you.

For 6 months, invest in yourself.

Begin today.

'Okay I'm down to take you up on this challenge. But bro, I'll be honest. I'm not too sure what investing in myself means.'

Gotcha, I'll explain my journey & you may get some ideas from that. Let's begin.

1. Cut off toxic people You become the energy that you surround yourself with. If you want to begin this 6-month journey, you need to distance yourself from people who aren't helping you grow.

2. **Take care of your body** I made it a priority to go to the gym, do yoga & play basketball.

-Gym for strength training.

-Yoga for flexibility & mental clarity.

-Basketball for fun & cardio.

Your body influences your mentality, so be sure to take care of it.

3. **Take care of your body part 2.**

'There's more??'

Yep.

-Eat healthy. Learn to cook!

-Stay hydrated.

-Get proper sleep.

4. **Mentality** I did the following to keep my mind sharp.

-Meditation

-Journaling (to organize my thoughts).

-Visualization with hype music (picture your best self & visualize that)

-Gratefulness exercises when I woke up & before I went to bed.

-Consumed empowering content.

5. **Emotional & spiritual clarity** I used these 6 months to get to know myself better. The main goal was to become my best friend. I made it a priority to get my alone time to get to know my inner world & my higher self. A lot of reflection & introspection.

6. **Built my circle from ground up** As I cut off negative people & built my life from ground up, something spectacular happened. I began attracting likeminded people. I used this stage to rebuild my squad full of winners & go getters.

7. **Production mode** This is the perfect opportunity to transition your life from a consumer to a producer. I spent time writing stories, giving speeches & building a side hustle. Find what works for you.

8. **Drop a bad habit & pick up a good habit** Self-explanatory, but this lifechanging. Remember, your habits dictate your reality, so make sure you're building the right neural pathways! Audit your habits & identify the negatives & find something positive to replace them with.

Now to be honest, I had no clue that I was going to be doing all of this. I just stumbled onto them as I began my journey. The best thing for you to do is the same. Just start & you will build your own path along the way.

6 months to change your life FOREVER? This is a no brainer.

Now enter the unknown & come back more powerful than ever!! Reality will never be the same.

Beautiful.

The Keys to Leveling Up

Your journal is your therapist.

Your mind is your mentor.

Your breath is your remote control.

Your awareness is your magnifying glass.

Let me go over each one. And be sure to pay attention VERY carefully. Each one is a massive tool for your level up journey.

•Your journal is your therapist.

The journal will have your back thru the thick & thin. No matter how bad life gets, your journal will stabilize you. Which is why you must write in it daily.

3 Ways to Journal:

1. Talk about your day.

2. Talk about your future.

3. Make sense of a painful life moment.

Journal Mind HACK:

If you still feel stiff with your writing, try this. Imagine that your present-day journals will one day be passed onto your kids. Write in a way so they can learn from your mistakes, experiences & life. You will feel more creative.

As the days fly by, journaling will become your therapy. You will notice:

-Clarity

-Emotional resiliency

-Stronger mind

•*Your mind is your mentor*

Your mind can become your mentor when you hack it. 'How do I hack it?' By creating an alter ego.

'How do I create an alter ego?'

Thru your imagination. Here's what you do:

1. Envision your ideal future self.

2. Give advice to your present-day self. When you do this, you'll unleash a new level of wisdom. Note: It is difficult before it is tactical.

Your mind is what you make it. If you think its power is limited, it will be limited. If you think its power is unlimited, it will be unlimited. Simple.

•Your breath is your remote control

Fast shallow breaths = Anxiety Slow deep breaths = Peace

Don't you see? Your breath was the remote control to your life all along. If you feel overly anxious, ANALYZE YOUR BREATH. Dial it to your whim. It is the gateway to your reality. Note: Meditation gives you the power to control your breath.

•Your awareness is your magnifying glass

You become what you focus on. You focus on what you put your awareness on.

Awareness is the invisible superpower of your mind. You can't see it. You can't touch it. But it is there.

Your awareness serves as your life's magnifying glass.

1. You can use it on yourself to identify overlooked flaws.

2. You can use it on yourself to shatter limiting beliefs.

3. You can use it to spot snakes. The powers are endless.

Want to know what's cool about all of these 4 elements? They allow you to level up from within.

-Your internal world creates your external world. Once you level up from within, the world around you begins to change. You begin to magnetize better people, opportunities & a boatload of abundance!

But most importantly, you feel CONFIDENT.

'I had the tools all along, huh?'

You absolutely did. Now go utilize them!

You will manifest your wildest desires.

Magic.

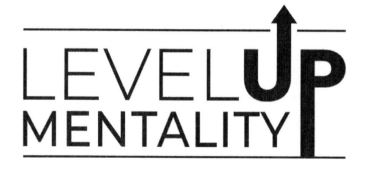

Bonus Part 2:

Cheat Codes & Mind Hacks

Cheat code to a better life

Sleep

I used to sleep on my sleep. Scraped a few hours a day. Bad move. Aim to get 7-8 hours. I get it, not easy in today's busy world. But make it an effort, and your production & happiness will skyrocket.

Meditate

Meditation has changed my life forever. I used to be this overthinking squirmy clown. But once you begin meditating routinely, life slows down, concentration improves, happiness improves & clarity improves. Do at least 10 minutes when waking up & 10 minutes before going to sleep.

Journal

Journaling is a game changer. You can do a word document or physical journal. Just get your thoughts & feelings written. Bonus: Do so every day and your writing skills will improve.

Visualize

I don't visualize like most people in silence. If I'm visualizing, I better have some lit music. Otherwise, it feels like work. My visualization routine has me envisioning positives AND negatives If it's a negative scenario I plan out my rise as well.

Do yoga

Seriously, do yoga. And no, it's not easy like you may think. Yoga allows you to synchronize your mind, breath & body. Very powerful. I use the yoga routine from p90x 3. But research a few routines from YouTube and see which one works best for you.

Financial literacy

You are not just born financially literate. Tame your ego & learn from books, ask questions to the right people, and become more curious. Learn this language inside & out.

Have hobbies

Major key. Life is going to kick your ass many times, make no mistake about that. Your hobbies will always keep you grounded even in your dark times. Have a hobby to keep you creative, one that makes you money & one that keeps you in shape.

Get sun

I'm not going to start giving you all these concepts on why sun is good for you. I just know ever since I have been going for a walk everyday outdoors, my life has improved. Go ahead and give it a try. Leave your dark room & Netflix binge session and get some sun.

Working out

This not only good for you physically, but mentally as well. To be honest, consistently showing dedication to your body is more mental than physical. Have a workout routine and stick to it.

Eat healthy

Put your twinkies & cup noodles away and take your fatass to the kitchen homie. Learn how to cook. Do not be dependent on fast food. Many view cooking as 'work' but not really. Learn a few dishes and you will realize it is fun. Recipes are everywhere online.

Drink water

Staying hydrated is very important. Proper hydration will have you thinking clearly & efficiently. However, do not overhydrate. Drinking too much water is just as bad as not drinking enough water. Use a water calculator online to find out your optimal level.

Have a social support system

Have friends & family you can count on. We are social creatures by blood. If you do not have a squad, go on and build one. People are not going to just break into your house asking to be your friend. Know when to work, know when to unwind.

Know when to rest

People think always working is a badge of honor. Not true! You need to rest. Otherwise, you risk burning out. You cannot run a smooth engine if it's always running. Learn to maintain your engine it by resting intelligently.

Cheat Code to Discipline: Working Out

Working out is one of the best ways to incorporate discipline into your life. Working out leads to eating right, sleeping well & structuring your day much better. If you have no clue how to be disciplined, start there.

'What does lifting a bunch of weights have to do with discipline?'

Tons. Working out is a life hack.

It is a life hack due to the chain effect of benefits that you get from it. Sparking the chain will have you unleashing a maximized disciplined effort towards life.

First, you need to fix your mindset towards the gym.

☆ Wrong: you go to the gym to work out your body.

☆ Right: you go to the gym to work out your mind & emotions, and an enhanced body is a side effect.

When you focus only on the body, you think short term. When you focus on the mind & emotions, you think lifelong.

What is discipline? Discipline is when your mind is capable of overriding disruptive emotions in order to follow a routine. Which is why disciplined people aren't chaotic creatures.

297

The disciplined person knows that they can feel disruptive emotions without having to succumb to it. They have a structure to always fall back on. The structure allows their mind & emotions to come into harmony.

Mind & Emotions in harmony leads to:

☆Happiness

☆Confidence

☆Productivity

This is why working out is important. Working out adds structure to your day. People who take care of their body know that working out doesn't stop at the gym. The gym is only scratching the surface. They also prep their meals, avoid sporadically spending money outdoors, play more sports, sleep well & all that.

Adding structure to your day helps you identify a bunch of the b.s activities that you were wasting your time on before. Now your life feels much more clarified because you got rid of the noise. Plus, you feel healthier & look better than ever.

People who think working out is only for the body are clearly just beginners. But people who have been doing it for a while, view it as more of a workout for their internal world.

Stick with it for long enough & you will view it to be the same. Working out is one of the most efficient ways to incorporate discipline into your life. Add discipline into one part & watch it positively spillover to other parts. Magic.

Cheat Code to Hack Wisdom:

Have elder mentors.

I don't care if they are in the same niche as you or not.

Their perspective will put you YEARS ahead of your time.

I always keep 5 elder mentors and am always searching for more to take me under their wing.

Level up at all times.

Cheat Code to Thick Skin:

1. Hype music

2. Envision situations where you are being tested

3. Envision tackling the challenges anyways

This method allows you to feel the exact emotions

Now when something bad happens in real life, the disruptive emotions will not throw you off

3 Ways to Hack Past Procrastination

1. Mindset- When you procrastinate, you are focusing too much on the big tasks. Stop, flip it. Focus on the small tasks & build up.

Ex: instead of focusing on getting the entire blog done, do 1 paragraph. You will strangely want to complete another paragraph...

2. Hype Song- Have one song that gets you hyped up. Promise yourself after playing the song 2-3 times, you will immediately begin. No questions asked, just begin.

The song amps up your emotions & you approach the task with energy.

3.Game- Turn mundane tasks into a game by using your creativity. If you're a gamer, break tasks into levels & kill each boss. If you like music, reward yourself with a song after each completion.

Challenge: Aim to do some pushups or pullups after each crossed off goal.

Mind Hack: 'Yet'

Anything that you do not have, but want, always finish it with 'yet.'

-I am not a millionaire....yet.

-My business has not taken off....yet.

-I have not reached my dream body....yet.

This hack will keep your mind searching for solutions. Remember:

-Words influence thoughts.

-Thoughts influence actions.

Therefore, adding in the one word of 'yet' does not terminate your desire. 'Yet' keeps the thought in open minded mode.

Ex: 'I am not an engineer.' This communicates to your primal mind that you are done-zo. But saying something like 'I am not an engineer...yet' allows you to still maintain your spirit.

Your spirit will drive your enthusiasm. Enthusiasm is needed for goal chasing.

So even if you do not have your desire yet, aim to still think correctly. Keep your mind in growth mode & watch your actions change completely. Very powerful & simple life hack. Go on & give it a try for your next desire.

Mind Hack: Replace 'problem' with 'challenge.'

When you say you have a problem, you feel a sense of defeat. When you say you have a challenge, you feel more optimistic to do something about it.

Let me clarify it with a Dragon Ball Z analogy.

In one of the seasons, there was a villain named Cell. Cell's power consisted of him absorbing other people from his tail & sucking all their energy. Cell strategically chose whose power he absorbed because he wanted to be as strong as possible.

The way that he was going to get power was absorbing the mighty characters, not the bums. Example of powerful characters: Android 17 & 18. Example of bums: Krillin & Yamcha. Who do you think Cell absorbed?

'The powerful ones!'

Exactly.

Well the same concept applies to your words. There are no shortages of words in the dictionary. Therefore, you have many options. You have the prerogative to choose words that have positive or negative energy. Completely up to you. Just know a few things.

1. Your words have energy that fuels or depletes your conscious mind.

2. Your subconscious mind hears everything.

Begin taking your words more seriously and experiment more. See which words have you feeling limited & which ones have you feeling unlimited.

Few recommendations:

-Replace 'problems' with 'challenges'

-Replace 'if' with 'when'

-Replace 'I have to' with 'I get to'

These are just 3 of many. Identify a few of your weak words today & see how you can flip the script! You'll be amazed.

You are the author of your story bud. Time to take more responsibility for how your life is playing out. Tick tock. Now go on & continue writing the greatest story ever.

Mind HACK: Days -> Opportunities

Start referring 'days' as 'opportunities.'

This mental shift has you approaching each day with more optimism.

Optimism paired with a clear purpose is deadly. You'll notice yourself crossing off your goals with more hunger & positive spirits.

Magic.

Mind HACK:
Replace 'I have to' with 'I get to.'

Example:

Wrong: I have to give a speech tonight.

Right: I get to give a speech tonight.

This hack gives your mind positive vibes & has you looking forward to the task.

Mind HACK: The Coach

Coach yourself.

Study how famous coaches operated.

Then be your own life coach.

Build your experiences & identify your strengths & weaknesses in the process.

This is a mind hack you can use to learn a new skillset or just your improve life in general.

Legend Building Hack

Put on your favorite hype music.

Now envision the grandest version of yourself.

Bigger. Bigger champ, you are not giving yourself enough credit.

Now make that even BIGGER.

Got it?

Now chase that vision until it becomes reality.

Trust me, it will.

Mind Hack: Phone Background

Change your phone background or laptop wallpaper to something that relates to your goal. Example: if you want to become a solid writer, have a picture of a book or something. This picture should make you feel. Remember, visuals & feelings talk to your subconscious mind.

Your subconscious mind dictates 95% of your reality? Your subconscious mind is the database & your conscious mind pulls the data from there. Which is why it is crucial to feed your subconscious mind empowering data.

The subconscious mind is like a little kid. It loves to see images, that make it feel. Your subconscious mind cannot tell the difference between what is imagined & what is real.

Which is why visualization is so important. You use your imagination to feed images to your subconscious mind. A changed subconscious mind is LIFECHANGING. Why? Because now your conscious mind is riding the waves of the tsunami rather than swimming against it.

Which ties back to the initial point, you are changing your background images because you are talking directly to the mind that dictates your future. Don't sleep on this trick. It will change your life.

But I want you to take it one level further. Get posters as well. So now you will wake up & go to sleep looking at your future. Find images that:

1. Relate to your goal.

2. Make you FEEL. (Important!)

And you are good to go.

You are in more control of your life than you have been giving yourself credit for. You are a lot more powerful than you have yet to realize. Now design the future you have been envisioning all along.

Mind Hack: Birthday Edition

My friend in college told me he read this strategy in a book or quote: But when identifying your age, use 'level' instead of 'years old.' Level tricks your mind into a growth mentality. I am level 27, each year is a gift, each year is a chance to level up.

Let me take it even a level further. I am going to explain why the 'years old' terminology is outdated and should be ditched. Believe it or not, 'years old' is detrimental in my eyes. Choose your words carefully. Here is why I would adopt 'level'

'Years old'

This terminology makes you a little scared to age. 'Oh my goodness, I am turning 30!' You think too physically. You view yourself as an aging product. Who the fuck wants to view themselves as that? Makes you think like you're a used car, getting worse with time.

That is why people are scared to age. They believe they are weakening. And to be honest, your body is aging, no fighting that. But what about your mind? Is your mind getting worse with time or better? If you are a victor, then it is exponentially getting better.

'Level'

Level tricks your focus back to your mind. You no longer view yourself as a used car that needs a Carfax report. Rather, you start making a mentality shift to 'aging like fine wine.' You now KNOW that you are getting better with time. You look forward to birthdays!

You've hacked the system. While everyone in society is using 'years old' because they were told to, you are being innovative. Small mental shifts add up like none other.

Adopt this strategy & your life will begin to change.

'So I won't ONLY be excited about birthdays? There's other side effects?'

Yep. The other side effect is that you are in growth mode year around. You want to keep leveling up your mind to new heights. Power.

Remember this. Your mind is your best friend in this life. The one with the strongest mind will always win. Start exercising your brain so your mentality aligns with your future goals.

Adopt the 'level' strategy & go on a conquest to grow. Separate yourself from the herd.

Life HACK: Laugh at your L's

Spend more time laughing at your mistakes after you make them.

This small hack has you rewiring your perception towards failures.

Try it out the next time you are picking up a new skillset.

Confidence Hack: Mirror Talking

1. Make direct eye contact with yourself in the mirror.

2. Speak your empowering thoughts into existence.

Every day, 15 minutes, 2 months.

After the 2 months you will:

-feel more comfortable in your own skin & surer of yourself.

'Can you explain why this hack works?'

Sure. Let me explain the 'why' so the 'what' makes a lot more sense. This is a life changing hack that will have you feeling more confident than ever. Confidence is your number 1 weapon in this world, so aim to fine tune it every. Read along:

Direct eye contact with the mirror does 2 things:

1. It allows you to work out your eye contact skills.

2. You see how you look when you are talking.

Many people think they look ugly when they talk. This is due to the 'illusion of transparency.'

Illusion of transparency is when you feel emotionally uncomfortable, so you think it is making you look ugly. You feel like the negative emotions is leaking out to the external world.

100% in your head. The mirror tactic conditions your mind to overpower the illusion of transparency. Results? You feel comfortable as fuck in your own skin.

So now you feel more confident & your eye contact skills have skyrocketed.

But why the empowering words? Subconscious reprogramming, my friend. That's why. There's a certain way I want you to speak for it to be the most effective for you.

Be **detailed** about your future. Use words that has you **feeling** something. You can't logically explain stuff to your subconscious mind. You need to hack it with visual images & emotion. So, speak powerful thoughts that has you feeling empowered. Rinse and repeat.

Keep doing this mirror strategy & you'll find yourself transforming into a new person. It worked for me & a few of the kids I used to mentor in Toastmasters. Very life changing. Go ahead and begin giving it a try. You seriously have nothing to lose. And guess what?

You become a better speaker as well! Begin today & take steps closer to compound gains.

Confidence Hack:
Take more trips by yourself.

This exercise allows you to connect with your internal world & get to know yourself better. Self-confidence is the truest form of confidence. Start planning something.

'Hmm interesting. Why does this hack work?'

For 2 Reasons:

1. Overcoming Self Consciousness.

2. A deeper understanding of self. Let me explain...

1. **Overcoming Self Consciousness** - A lot of people are unable to take trips by themselves. They think it's 'weird' to do it. And they feel embarrassed for not having someone to take a trip with. Heck, you may fall into this boat right now.

How often have you canceled a trip or event because people flaked?

'Too many times to count.'

Why?

'Because going by myself would feel awkward.'

Why?

'Because I need to go with people.'

No, you don't. That's a limiting belief.

Confidence is when it's good to have people around you, but you are not dependent on them. You can make your own moves as you please. Going on a few trips by yourself transitions your mind from:

-Dependent -> Independent.

2. **A deeper understanding of self** - Believe it or not, you'll come out of a trip with more clarity. You have the chance to spend time with yourself in a new environment. Currently, you don't have the responsibilities, bills & problems of the real world consuming your mind.

This frees your mind to reflect on other things. Making sense of your past, finding clarity on the present, architecting a structure for your future. As long as you aren't on your phone all day, you will come out with a deeper sense of self.

This hack may seem very unorthodox, but it works. Before ruling it off, give it a try. Find a weekend where you can go somewhere new. Go by yourself & restrict technology usage. Now just explore & reflect!

This weekend trip will have a bigger impact on your future than you can possibly imagine. Give it a try & grasp control of your internal world!

Mind Hack:
Motivational Videos

Motivational videos without the work is like listening to gym music without going to the gym.

But combining motivational videos WITH work is a HACK.

Those videos charge up your emotions & have you imagining.

-Subconscious rewiring 101.

Use it as a tool for your journey.

Mind Hack: Destination -> Journey

Ditch the 'destination' mentality.

Adopt the 'journey' mentality.

This mind shift allows you to focus more on perfecting the process rather than just focusing on the end goal.

Get it?

Perfect the process & the end goal is guaranteed.

Mind HACK:
Focus Sharpeners

View boring tasks as 'focus sharpeners'

-doing the dishes

-folding laundry

-cleaning your room

Exercising your focus in one area of your life spills over to other parts .

While everyone is doing these tasks with negativity, you're doing it to level up your mind.

Wisdom HACK: Tweet advice to your 5-year-old self

Adopting this perspective will give you a higher authority mindset while maintaining an informal tone. You will start dropping wisdom that you never knew existed within you.

This hack works so well because of 2 big principles:

1. Authority

2. Informality

1. **Authority** The reason I say choose your 5-year-old self is because you maintain a sense of responsibility. You will avoid giving wreck less advice because you are an authority figure. This helps you adopt a different perspective.

2. **Informality** An informal mindset breeds creativity. And creativity will help you approach your advice with more angles than you previously thought of.

'I see. But why tweet it?'

That's just a suggestion. You will notice as you are tweeting advice to your younger self, it will resonate with a lot of people from around the world. So not only are helping yourself, but you're helping others along the way. 2 birds, 1 stone.

But other avenues to give advice to your younger self are thru:

-Journaling

-Podcasting

One will help you with your writing. The other will help you with your speaking.

Plus, this is the most important part of this trick.. Giving advice to your younger self is a subtle way to reprogram your mindset! Your subconscious mind is like a little kid, so it listens carefully when you talk to it like a little kid.

'So I gain wisdom, help people AND rewire my mindset?'

Correct! Give this life hack a try today & put yourself ahead of the herd.

3 Victim Mentality Busters:

-Accountability for ALL of life's conflicts. You will rise regardless.

-Improve body language. Your body effects the mind.

-Read some fiction. Rewire your brain to think big.

Productivity HACK:

Before work on something that requires intense focus, do a meditation session beforehand.

Count your natural breaths to 50.

Doing this alone will skyrocket your production.

Productivity Hack:

If you are working from home, dress up & wear shoes too.

This hacks your subconscious into a productive state of mind.

Afterward

I would like to thank you for making it to the end of the book. First, I would like to say thank you for investing your time for reading this material. A lot of the content from this book is created from a ton of hardships, failures & introspection. If the concepts & teaching in this book can help one person, then it has served its purpose.

Also, I would like to thank my parents who have been supportive of me in my journey. They have made a lot of sacrifices for me to be in this country & become an engineer. Their contributions have played a big factor in me being able to become an author. I would also like to thank my older brother for always having my back & helping me stay on track.

A person's social circle will play a great deal in their reality. There have been plenty of friends that have contributed to this book, too many to name. Thus far, I have had the opportunity to make real life & digital connections. In real life, I met a lot of winners from Toastmasters, the city of Tampa, clubs, conferences etc. And I have made a lot of digital connections thru Twitter, YouTube & my website.

I hope you apply the concepts in the book & turn your life around for the best. We are given only one opportunity in this life & the ability to sculpt our future is what will allow us to gain power in this volatile world. Even if you are feeling lost right now, understand it's never too late. Now take the time & re-engineer your mindset towards confidence so you can become your grandest self.

To find more of my content, head over to www.armanitalks.com, where you will see plenty of my blogs, podcasts & videos helping you use 5 soft skills to level up your confidence: public speaking, storytelling, emotional intelligence, social dynamics & creativity. Thanks again for reading!

- **ARMANI**TALKS 🎙️🔥

Printed in Great Britain
by Amazon